Physiological Responses to Intermittent Hypoxia in Humans

by

Jon C. Kolb

ISBN: 1-58112-241-1

DISSERTATION.COM

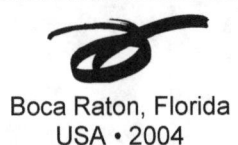

Boca Raton, Florida
USA • 2004

Physiological Responses to Intermittent Hypoxia in Humans

Dissertation.com
Boca Raton, Florida
USA • 2004

ISBN: 1-58112-241-1

PHYSIOLOGICAL RESPONSES

TO INTERMITTENT HYPOXIA IN HUMANS

By

Jon C. Kolb

A Thesis

Submitted to the Institute for the Theory and Practice of Training

and Movement, German Sport University Cologne.

October, 2003

TABLE OF CONTENTS

LIST OF FIGURES

LIST OF TABLES

CHAPTER 1

INTRODUCTION

1.1   INTRODUCTION

Hypoxia is a general reduction in oxygen delivery, either because of decreased arterial oxygen content, decreased cardiac output, or decreased oxygen uptake in the systemic capillaries, which may result from a multitude of medical complications, environmental factors, or physical exertion. The complex physiologic and symptomatic adaptations to hypoxia have been extensively investigated during the past century (Bert, 1878; FitzGerald, 1914; Pugh, 1964; Roach and Hackett, 2001; Basnyat and Murdoch; 2003). Interest in the effects of hypoxia is of clinical importance in determining the pathophysiology of cerebrovascular diseases (Schoene, 1999; Segler, 2001; Severinghaus, 2001) and cardiopulmonary diseases (Neubauer, 2001; Morgan and Joyner, 2002; Serebrovskaya, 2002). Furthermore, understanding the adaptive changes which occur during high altitude sojourns is physiologically relevant in discerning the etiology of diseases such as acute mountain sickness and high altitude cerebral edema (Hackett et al., 1998). From an applied point of view, sport physiologists have for many years investigated the potential ergogenic benefits of altitude training and subsequent improvement in athletic performance (Buskirk et al., 1967; Faulkner et al., 1967; Wilbur, 2001; Levine, 2002).

1.1.1   Acclimatization to Hypoxia

Acclimatization to chronic hypoxia follows a time dependent continuum (minutes, days, weeks) which progresses through increased ventilation, alterations in cerebrovascular and cardiovascular dynamics, and subsequently metabolic changes at the tissue level which reciprocally function to enhance oxygen extraction and utilization (Hackett, 2002). Acute hypoxia is detected by the carotid bodies located close to the bifurcation of the common carotid artery. The high rate of perfusion in the carotid body combined with its' sensitivity to a reduction in the partial pressure of oxygen, activates afferent impulses to the respiratory center of the medulla stimulating an increase in pulmonary ventilation (Dempsey and Forster, 1982; Smith et al., 1986; Lahiri et al., 2000). Hypocapnia and respiratory alkalosis occur secondary following this hypoxic-induced ventilatory stimuli (Moore et al., 1986; Weil, 1986). While hypocapnia alone normally results in cerebral vasoconstriction, the effect is significantly offset by reduced oxygen delivery to the brain at altitude, resulting in a net decline in cerebral vascular resistance and a reciprocal increase in cerebral blood flow (Otis et al., 1989; Krasney, 1994; Buck et al., 1998; Jansen et al., 1999; Severinghaus, 2001).

Similarly, increased heart rate, reduced plasma volume, and elevated hematocrit work synergistically to optimize the circulatory function assisting oxygenation at the tissue level. Erythropoietin, released from the hypoxic kidney, increases red blood cell mass overtime further enhancing oxygen delivery to the cell in an attempt to regain homeostasis (Milledge and Cotes, 1985; Eckardt et al., 1989). With respect to high altitude physiology and the numerous ventilatory and hematological changes associated with hypoxic stress, several authors have reported a relationship between the degree of hypoxemia and the onset of acute mountain sickness (AMS) (Roach et al., 1998; Saito et al., 1999; Hussain et al., 2001; Kolb et al., 2001). Symptoms associated with AMS include headache, lethargy, fatigue, peripheral edema, and loss of appetite (Singh et al., 1969; Hackett and Rennie, 1976). The pathology of AMS follows a complex symptomatic continuum, the severity of which is dependent on altitude gained, rate of ascent, prior acclimatization, and the individual's susceptibility to the effects of lowered arterial oxygen concentration (Lyons et al., 1995; Powell and Garcia, 2000; Roach and Hackett, 2001).

Although the physiological responses to hypoxia are extensive, this dissertation focuses specifically on alterations in both respiratory control and cerebrovascular responses. Vasomotor reactivity to acute hypoxia has been suggested by several authors to trigger cerebral vasodilation and hence cerebral blood flow (CBF), which may in turn initiate the clinical symptoms of AMS (Krasney, 1994; Jansen et al., 1999; Schoene, 1999). If the hypoxic stress is severe and continuous, cerebral edema may develop, and in some individuals may progress to high altitude cerebral edema (HACE) characterized by ataxia and altered levels of consciousness (Hackett, 1999a).

A recent review of cerebral circulation at high altitude (Severinghaus, 2001) identified that individual variability in the magnitude of cerebral blood flow changes in response to hypoxia depends on the integrated drive of four reflexive mechanisms:

   i.   The acute ventilatory response to hypoxia (AHVR).

   ii.   The acute ventilatory response to increased arterial carbon dioxide (AHCVR).

   iii.   The cerebral vasodilative response to hypoxia.

   iv.   The cerebral vasoconstrictive response associated with hypocapnia.

The array of complex interactions between ventilatory and cerebrovascular systems during periods of reduced oxygenation has potential implications on virtually all major physiological systems. Therefore the remainder of this chapter considers specific alterations in AHVR, AHCVR, and the cerebrovascular responses to hypoxemia.

1.1.2   Ventilatory Acclimatization to Hypoxia

The sensitivity of the carotid bodies to reductions in arterial oxygen pressure (PaO_2) governs the extent to which AHVR is augmented (Smith et al., 1986). An increase in the AHVR allows ventilatory acclimatization to proceed, despite respiratory alkalosis and a withdrawal of the stimulus to the peripheral chemoreceptors (Dempsey and Forster, 1982). Similarly an increase in the

AHCVR occurs during chronic hypoxia as the central chemorecptors respond to reduced end-tidal P_{CO_2} (Cunningham et al., 1986).

As a diagnostic tool, AHVR by definition is an assessment of an individuals ventilatory sensitivity to progressive isocapnic hypoxia (Ward et al., 2000). Historically, methods for measuring ventilatory sensitivities to hypoxia have included brief exposures (five to ten minutes) of progressively reduced inspiratory oxygen content (Weil et al., 1970) or re-breathing methods that generate a hypoxic stimulus (Rebuck and Campbell, 1974) in which the end tidal carbon dioxide pressure ($P_{ET_{CO_2}}$) is held constant (isocapnic). The isocapnic control throughout the test is important to isolate the ventilatory drive associated with hypoxia, which would otherwise be masked by the reduction in CO_2 as a result of hyperventilation and therefore reduce the stimulus to breath (Grover, 1994). Both methods (Weil et al., 1970; Rebuck and Campbell, 1974) quantify AHVR by comparing ventilation to end tidal oxygen pressure ($P_{ET_{O_2}}$). More recently, progressive isocapnic hypoxic protocols have been used to describe AHVR by comparing the ratio of changes in ventilation with changes in SaO_2 (Mou et al., 1995; Katayama et al., 1999). Alternatively, a series of square wave pulses of hypoxia, where carbon dioxide levels were fixed at the subjects resting level, has been utilized in accurately quantifying AHVR through a mathematical fitting model that incorporates both peripheral and central chemoreflexes (Howard and Robbins, 1995). The model developed by a group from the University of Oxford, describes parameter G_p (hypoxic sensitivity), which represents the change in ventilation for a given change in SaO_2.

Regardless of the methodology used, several investigators have reported that AHVR increases following relatively short (eight hours) exposures to hypoxia (Howard and Robbins, 1995; Fatemian et al., 2001) days or weeks of hypoxia (Schoene et al., 1990; Tansley et al., 1998), and that elevated ventilatory responses to hypoxia may persist for up to a week following hypoxic conditioning (Katayama et al., 1999). As such, the increases in AHVR which arises from hypoxia elevates SaO_2 improving oxygenation, and therefore has been identified as a cornerstone of ventilatory acclimatization (Casas et al., 2000). However, between-individual AHVR variation is great, and a blunted HVR may contribute to the suseptabilty of AMS via attenuation of the arterial oxygen content (Schoene, 1982; Moore et al., 1986; Matsuzawa et al., 1989; Casas et al., 2000; Bartsch et al., 2001).

1.1.3   Cerebrovascular Responses to Hypoxia

1.1.3.1   Cerebral Blood Flow
Over fifty years ago reduced inspired oxygen fraction ($F_iO_2 = 0.10$) was reported to result in an SaO_2 of 65% in humans, while cerebral blood flow (CBF) determined from N_2O uptake by the brain, exhibited an increase of 35% when compared to resting ventilation under normoxic conditions (Kety and Schmidt, 1948). The first measurement of human CBF response to high altitude (3810m)

using the methodology of Kety and Schmidt (Kety and Schmidt, 1945) indicated a 24% increase over sea level values (Severinghaus et al., 1966). More recently, the non-invasive technique of transcranial Doppler ultrasonography (TCD) has been employed for the accurate evaluation of cerebral blood flow in response to acute variations in O_2 and CO_2 (Poulin et al., 1996; Poulin et al., 2002).

Using TCD to determine the velocity of cerebral blood flow (CBFv), stepwise acute isocapnic hypoxia ($SaO_2 \cong$ 90, 80, 70, 60%) resulted in a 35% increase in normal human subjects residing at sea level (Jensen et al., 1996). Interestingly, after five days of altitude acclimatization (3810m), the same subjects exhibited a 46% increase in CBFv to the stepwise isocapnic hypoxia test, thus indicating an increased cerebral vasoreactivity following five days of continuous hypoxia. Jensen and colleagues (1996) identified a hyperbolic association between CBFv and SaO_2, similar in shape to AHVR.

Middle cerebral artery velocity (MCAv) was measured in climbers ascending to high altitude to assess the relationship between CBF regulation and the onset of AMS (Otis et al., 1989). Using TCD, a significant increase in MCAv was noted between sea level control values and measurements obtained at 4115m (55 ± 7 and 71 ± 13cm/sec respectively). Otis and colleagues (1989) suggested that the increased CBF in theory may contribute to the pathophysiology of AMS and HACE due to a transcranial leakage from increased arterial blood pressure resulting in cerebral edema and increased inctracranial pressure leading to displacement and stretching of the pain sensitive trigeminovascular structures. This 'vasogenic theory', associated with high altitude headache, AMS, and HACE has since been supported by several research groups (Krasney, 1994; Buck et al., 1998; Hackett, 1999b; Sanchez del Rio and Moskowita, 1999).

Similarly, following 72 hours at an elevation of 4559m, MCAv (quantified by TCD) and blood gas analysis of arterial PO_2 were measured in concert with self reported AMS symptomatology in 23 healthy males (Baumgartner et al., 1994). The mean cerebral blood velocity increased 148 ± 16% over sea level values in subjects reporting AMS, while the increase was 127 ± 24% in subjects without AMS. Baumgartner and colleagues (1994) also identified that MCAv exhibited a significant negative correlation (r = -0.51, p < 0.001) with arterial PO_2 throughout the high altitude exposure.

Further evidence that increased cerebral vasomotor reactivity contributes to the development of AMS has been described in high altitude trekkers reaching Pheriche (4243m) en route to Mount Everest Base Camp (Jansen et al., 1999). The Lake Louise AMS scoring system questionnaire (Roach et al., 1993) was employed to classify the climbers into two groups: those presenting with AMS symptoms and subjects reporting no AMS. Data collected by Jansen's group (1999) included TCD quantification of MCAv, SaO_2, and transcutaneous PCO_2. While PCO_2 levels were essentially the same, subjects exhibiting AMS symptoms had higher resting cerebral blood velocity than did no AMS subjects (74 ± 22 and 56 ± 14cm/s respectively). Additionally, SaO_2 was significantly lower in AMS subjects compared to no AMS subjects ($80 \pm 8\%$ and $88 \pm 3\%$ respectively).

1.1.3.2 Cerebral Oxygenation

The non-invasive assessment of cerebral oxygenation with near infrared spectroscopy was first described in 1991 (McCormick et al., 1991) as a new monitoring index to estimate cerebral regional oxygen saturation (S_rO_2).

Method comparison validation studies have illustrated the accuracy of cerebral oximetry (Grubhofer et al., 1999; Kim et al., 2000; Shah et al., 2000) while a number of publications have identified various clinical applications (Blas et al., 1999; Higami et al., 1999; Yao et al., 2001) as well as the utility in determining exercise intensity in humans (Nielsen et al., 1999; Saito et al., 1999).

Cerebral oximetry has also been employed to assess the oxygen status of the brain during sojourns to high altitude (Imray et al., 1998). Sea level cerebral oxygenation measurements were made on male (17) and female (3) volunteers with a Critikon 2020 cerebral oximeter (Johnson and Johnson Medical Ltd., UK) and following rapid ascent by automobile to 2270, 3650, and 4680m on consecutive days. In this, the first reported investigation monitoring cerebral oxygenation in the field at altitude, Imray and colleagues (1998) reported a parallel decline in both SaO_2 and S_rO_2, while AMS symptoms, diagnosed with the

Lake Louise AMS scoring system questionnaire (Roach et al., 1993), were more severe as SrO_2 fell (r = -0.41, p >0.05<0.1). As well, cerebral deoxygenation has been observed in unacclimatized trekkers at altitude (4300m) (Saito et al., 1999). Saito and colleagues (1999) suggest that the acute reduction in S_rO_2, followed by increased CBF, might be a primary cause of headache and AMS. Thus, the non-invasive monitoring of cerebral oxygenation is likely to be of critical importance in determining physiologic and symptomatic function at high altitude.

1.1.4   Intermittent Hypoxia

While much is known about the physiological responses to acute and chronic hypoxic exposures, far less is known about the effects of intermittent hypoxia (Powell and Garcia, 2000; Schmidt, 2002). Intermittent hypoxia, also referred to as discontinuous hypoxia, has been defined as repeated exposures to hypoxia, which are separated by periods of normoxia, or by episodes of hypoxia that are less severe (Powell and Garcia, 2000; Neubauer, 2001). Intermittent hypoxic protocols utilized with human subjects have varied greatly with respect to the total time frame of episodic cycles, the severity of hypoxia, and the number of hypoxic cycles per day. Relatively short protocols have varied from those that examined alternating between five minutes of hypoxia (simulated altitude of 6,000m) and five minutes of normoxia over sixty minutes twice per day for sixty days (Hellemans, 1999), to protocols which investigated ninety minutes of hypoxia (simulated altitudes of 4000m and 5500m) three times per week for 3 weeks

(Rodriguez et al., 2000). Extended discontinuous hypoxic protocols have incorporated eight to ten hours of overnight hypoxia for twenty-one days (Townsend et al., 2002) or longer cycles (twelve to sixteen hours per day) of hypoxia (simulated altitude, 2500m) over a twenty-five day period (Rusko et al., 1999). Irrespective of the protocol design, these repeated hypoxic episodes separated by periods of normoxia, have elicited changes in respiratory control (Rodriguez et al., 2000; Townsend et al., 2002) and hematogenesis (Hellemans, 1999; Rodriguez et al., 2000; Townsend et al., 2002), suggesting that there may be a cumulative effect of intermittent hypoxic episodes (Neubauer, 2001). Whether or not similar mechanisms are responsible for the physiological adaptations to discontinuous bouts of hypoxia are the same as those observed during chronic hypoxia, remains to be established (Powell and Garcia, 2000).

Recently, endurance athletes and high altitude climbers have gained access to commercially available, portable normobaric hypoxic chambers. Intermittent exposures to hypoxia in these chambers may elicit adaptations similar to those observed during acclimatization to altitude (Wilbur, 2001; Schmidt, 2002). Manufactures of these systems purport that intermittent exposures may elicit adaptations similar to those observed in response to the hypoxia of high altitude, however there have been no reports in the scientific literature that ventilatory acclimatization or alterations in cerebrovascular dynamics occur following repeated episodes in the portable chambers.

Thus, the goal of this dissertation is to provide a detailed investigation into the physiologic and symptomatic responses following an intervention of discontinuous normobaric hypoxia, which employs portable chambers. To accomplish this, an intermittent protocol was developed which cycled between 8 hrs of nocturnal hypoxia at a simulated altitude of 4300m, followed by 16 hrs of normoxia, for five consecutive days. Specifically, it is not currently known if cerebrovascular and ventilatory sensitivities to acute hypoxia are altered, or if altitude-like symptoms develop, in response to such an intermittent hypoxic protocol. This understanding will contribute to the emerging body of knowledge concerning dose-response effects owing to intermittent hypoxia, in determining whether the responses elicit protective adaptations, or cross over the dosage threshold, resulting in pathological disorders.

1.2 OBJECTIVES OF THESIS

Using normobaric hypoxia to elicit various levels of hypoxemia in humans, the following objectives are outlined to show the logical progression of experiments designed to engender a better understanding of changes in respiratory control and cerebrovascular dynamics following intermittent hypoxia:

1) Determine the validity of pulse oximetry in monitoring the state of arterial oxygenation during progressive normobaric hypoxia.

2) Develop a protocol for quantifying the cerebrovascular and ventilatory responses to acute variations in oxygen and carbon dioxide.

3) Design and implement a discontinuous hypoxic intervention to determine the extent and time frame for the development, and reversibility, of physiological and symptomatic perturbations.

It is envisaged that accomplishing these objectives will lead to a greater understanding of the dose-response effect of discontinuous hypoxia, and will provide insight regarding the basic efficacy of intermittent hypoxia. Specific aims and hypotheses are outlined in each respective chapter.

1.3   STRUCTURE OF THESIS AND PRESENTATION

The studies within the thesis are separated into four distinct phases, which were conducted sequentially. This sequential construction of the thesis was necessary because the results of each phase helped to finalize the research protocol for each subsequent investigation. Presentation of the dissertation is carried out as follows: Chapters 2, 3 , 4, and 5 are based on manuscripts that have been accepted

for publication in peer reviewed journals (i.e. Chapters 2 and 4), or are currently
under review Chapters 3 and 5), which fulfill the three objectives outlined in the
previous section. Chapter 6 concludes with a general discussion of the results
along with suggestions for future research. Chapters 2 through 5 each contain a
brief review of pertinent literature, details of methods and results, and a focused
discussion.

1.4 REFERENCES

Bartsch, P., Grunig, E., Hohenhaus, E. and Dehnert, C. (2001). Assessment of high altitude tolerance in healthy individuals. High Altitude Medicine & Biology 2(2): 287-96.

Basnyat, B. and Murdoch, D. R. (2003). High altitude illness. Lanct. 361(9373): 1967-74.

Baumgartner, R. W., Bartsch, P., Maggiorini, M., Waber, U. and Oelz, O. (1994). Enhanced cerebral blood flow in acute mountain sickness. Aviation Space & Environmental Medicine 65(8): 726-729.

Bert, P. (1878). La pression barometrique. Recherches de physiologie experiments. 1168 p. Paris, G. Mason

Blas, M., Sulek, C., Martin, T. and Lobato, E. (1999). Use of near-infrared spectroscopy to Monitor cerebral oxygenation during coronary artery bypass in a patient with bilateral internal carotid artery occlusion. Journal of Cardiothoracic and vascular anesthesia 13(6): 732-735.

Buck, A., Schirlo, C., Jasinksy, V., Weber, B., Burger, C., von Schulthess, G. K., Koller, E. A. and Pavlicek, V. (1998). Changes of cerebral blood flow during short-term exposure to normobaric hypoxia. Journal of Cerebral Blood Flow & Metabolism 18(8): 906-10.

Buskirk, E. R., Kollias, J., Akers, F., Prokop, E. K. and Reategui, E. P. (1967). Maximal performance at altitude and return from altitude in conditioned runners. Journal of Applied Physiology 23: 259-266.

Casas, M., Casas, H., Pages, T., Rama, R., Ricart, A., Ventura, J. L., Ibanez, J., Rodriguez, F. A. and Viscor, G. (2000). Intermittent hypobaric hypoxia induces altitude acclimation and improves the lactate threshold. Aviation Space & Environmental Medicine 71(2): 125-30.

Cunnningham, D.J.C., Robbins, P.A., and Wolf, C.B. (1986). Integration of respiratory responses to changes in alveolar partial pressures of CO_2 and O_2 and in arterial pH. In: Fishman, A.P. Handbook of Physiology, Section 3: The Respiratory System, Vol. II, Part 2: Control of Breathing. American Physiology Society, Bethesda, MD, pp. 475-528.

Dempsey, J.A., and Forster, H.V. (1982). Mediation of ventilatory adaptations. Physiological Reviews 62, 262-346.

Eckardt, K. U., Boutellier, U., Kurtz, A., Schopen, M., Koller, E. A. and Bauer, C. (1989). Rate of erythropoietin formation in humans in response to acute hypobaric hypoxia. Journal of Applied Physiology 66(4): 1785-8.

Fatemian, M., Kim, D. Y., Poulin, M. J. and Robbins, P. A. (2001). Very mild exposure to hypoxia for 8 h can induce ventilatory acclimatization in humans. Pflugers Archiv - European Journal of Physiology 441(6): 840-3.

Faulkner, J. A., Daniels, J. T. and Balke, B. (1967). Effects of training at moderate altitude on physical performance capacity. Journal of Applied Physiology 23: 85-89.

FitzGerald, M. P. (1914). Further observations on the changes in the breathing and the blood at various high altitudes. Proceedings of the Royal Society of London. Series B, Containing Papers of a Biological Character. 88(602): 248-258.

Grover, R. F. (1994). To breathe or not to breathe. Journal of Wilderness Medicine 5: 251-253.

Grubhofer, W., Tonninger, W., Keznickl, P., Skyllouriotis, P., Ehrlich, M., Hiesmayr, M. and Lassnigg, A. (1999). A comparison of the monitors INVOS 3100 and NIRO 500 in detecting changes in cerebral oxygenation. Acta Anaesthesiologica Scandinavica 43: 470-475.

Hackett, P. H. (1999a). The cerebral etiology of high-altitude cerebral edema and acute mountain sickness. Wilderness & Environmental Medicine 10(2): 97-109.

Hackett, P. H. (1999b). High altitude cerebral edema and acute mountain sickness. A pathophysiology update. Advances in Experimental Medicine & Biology 474: 23-45.

Hackett, P. H. (2002). High altitude medicine. *In: Wilderness Medicine: Management of Wilderness and Environmental Emergencies*. P. Auerbach. St. Louis, MO, CV Mosby: 2-43.

Hackett, P. H. and Rennie, D. (1976). The incidence, importance, and prophylaxis of acute mountain sickness. *Lancet* 2(7996): 1149-55.

Hackett, P. H., Yarnell, P. R., Hill, R., Reynard, K., Heit, J. and McCormick, J. (1998). High-altitude cerebral edema evaluated with magnetic resonance imaging: clinical correlation and pathophysiology. Journal of the American Medical Association 280(22): 1920-5.

Hellemans, J. (1999). Intermittent hypoxic training: a pilot study. Proceedings of the Second Annual International Altitude Training Symposium; 1999 Feb 18-20; Flagstaff (AZ): 145-154.

Higami, T., Kozawa, S., Asada, T., Obo, H., Gan, K., Iwahashi, K. and Nohara, H. (1999). Retrograde cerebral perfusion versus selective cerebral perfusion as evaluated by cerebral oxygen saturation during aortic arch reconstruction. Annals of Thoracic Surgery 67: 1091-1096.

Houston, C. S., Sutton, J. R., Cymerman, A. and Reeves, J. T. (1987). Operation Everest II: man at extreme altitude. Journal of Applied Physiology. 63(2): 877-82.

Howard, L. S. and Robbins, P. A. (1995). Alterations in respiratory control during 8 h of isocapnic and poikilocapnic hypoxia in humans. Journal of Applied Physiology 78(3): 1098-107.

Hussain, M. M., Aslam, M. and Khan, Z. (2001). Acute mountain sickness score and hypoxemia. Journal of the Pakistan Medical Association 51(5): 173-179.

Ide, K. and Secher, N. H. (2000). Cerebral blood flow and metabolism during exercise. Progress in Neurobiology 61: 397-414.

Imray, C. H. E., Barnett, N. J., Walsh, S., Clarke, T., Morgan, J., Hale, D., Hoar, H., Mole, D., Chesner, I. and Wright, A. D. (1998). Near-infrared spectroscopy in the assessment of cerebral oxygenation at high altitude. Wilderness & Environmental Medicine 9: 198-203.

Jansen, G. F., Krins, A. and Basnyat, B. (1999). Cerebral vasomotor reactivity at high altitude in humans. Journal of Applied Physiology 86(2): 681-6.

Jensen, J. B., Sperling, B., Severinghaus, J. W. and Lassen, N. A. (1996). Augmented hypoxic cerebral vasodilation in men during 5 days at 3,810 m altitude. Journal of Applied Physiology 80(4): 1214-8.

Katayama, K., Sato, Y., Morotome, Y., Shima, N., Ishida, K., Mori, S. and Miyamura, M. (1999). Ventilatory chemosensitive adaptations to intermittent hypoxic exposure with endurance training and detraining. Journal of Applied Physiology 86(6): 1805-11.

Kety, S. S. and Schmidt, C. F. (1945). The determination of cerebral blood flow in man by the use of nitrous oxide in low concentrations. American Journal of Physiology 143: 53-66.

Kety, S. S. and Schmidt, C. F. (1948). The effects of altered arterial tensions of carbon dioxide and oxygen on cerebral blood flow and cerebral oxygen consumption of normal young men. Journal of Clinical Investigation 27: 484-492.

Kim, M. B., Ward, D. S., Cartwright, C. R., Kolano, J., Chelhowski, S. and Henson, L. C. (2000). Estimation of Jugular Venous O_2 Saqturation from cerebral oximetry or arterial O_2 saturation during isocapnic hypoxia. Journal of Clinical Monitoring 16: 191-199.

Kolb, J., Norris, S., Smith, D., Henderson, J. and Hillis, F. (2001). Intermittent normobaric hypoxia enhances acclimation. High Altitude Medicine & Biology 2(1): 109.

Krasney, J. A. (1994). A neurogenic basis for acute altitude illness. Medicine & Science in Sports & Exercise 26(2): 195-208.

Lahiri, S., Rozanov, C., and Cherniack, N. S. (2000). Altered structure of the carotid body at high altitude and associated chemoreflexes. High Altitude Medicine & Biology 1: 63-74.

Levine, B. D. (2002). Intermittent hypoxic training: Fact or fancy. High Altitude Medicine & Biology 3: 177-193.

Lyons, T. P., Muza, S. R., Rock, P. B. and Cymerman, A. (1995). The effect of altitude pre-acclimatization on acute mountain sickness during reexposure. Aviation Space and Environmental Medicine 66(10): 957-962.

Matsuzawa, Y., Fujimoto, K., Kobayashi, T., Namushi, N. R., Harada, K., Kohno, H., Fukushima, M. and Kusama, S. (1989). Blunted hypoxic ventilatory drive in subjects susceptible to high-altitude pulmonary edema. Journal of Applied Physiology 66(3): 1152-7.

McCormick, P. W., Stewart, M., Goetting, M. G. and Balakrishnam, G. (1991). Regional cerebrovascular oxygen saturation by optical spectroscopy in humans. Stroke 22: 596-602.

Milledge, J. S. and Cotes, P. M. (1985). Serum erythropoietin in humans at high altitude and its relation to plasma renin. Journal of Applied Physiology 59(2): 360-4.

Moore, L. G., Harrison, G. L., McCullough, R. E., McCullough, R. G., Micco, A. J., Tucker, A., Weil, J. V. and Reeves, J. T. (1986). Low acute hypoxic ventilatory response and hypoxic depression in acute altitude sickness. Journal of Applied Physiology 60(4): 1407-12.

Morgan, B. J. and Joyner, M. J. (2002). Sleep apnea: A new 'risk factor' for cardiovascular disease. Exercise and Sport Sciences Reviews: 145-146.

Mou, X. B., Howard, L. S. and Robbins, P. A. (1995). A protocol for determining the shape of the ventilatory response to hypoxia in humans. Respiration Physiology 101(2): 139-43.

Neubauer, J. (2001). Physiological and pathophysiological responses to intermittent hypoxia. Journal of Applied Physiology 90: 1593-1599.

Nielsen, H. B., Boushel, R., Madsen, P. and Secher, N. H. (1999). Cerebral desaturation during exercise reversed by O_2 supplementation. American Journal of Physiology 277(Heart Circ. Physiol. 46): H1045-H1052.

Otis, S. M., Rossman, M. E., Schneider, P. A., Rush, M. P. and Ringelstein, E. B. (1989). Relationship of cerebral blood flow regulation to acute mountain sickness. Journal of Ultrasound in Medicine 8(3): 143-8.

Owen-Reece, H., Smith, M., Elwell, C. E. and Goldstone, J. C. (1999). Near infrared spectroscopy. British Journal of Anaesthesia 82(3): 418-426.

Poulin, M. J., Fatemian, M., Tansley, J. G., O'Connor, D. F. and Robbins, P. A. (2002). Changes in cerebral blood flow during and after 48 h of both isocapnic and poikilocapnic hypoxia in humans. Experimental Physiology 87.5: 633-642.

Poulin, M. J., Liang, P. J. and Robbins, P. A. (1996). Dynamics of the cerebral blood flow response to step changes in end-tidal PCO_2 and PO_2 in humans. Journal of Applied Physiology 81(3): 1084-1095.

Powell, F. L. and Garcia, N. (2000). Physiological effects of intermittent hypoxia. High Altitude Medicine & Biology 1(2): 125-136.

Pugh, G. (1964). Cardia output in muscular exercise at 5800m (19,000ft). Journal of Applied Physiology 19(3): 441-447.

Rebuck, A. S. and Campbell, E. J. M. (1974). A clinical method for assessing the ventilatory response to hypoxia. American Review of Respiratory Disease 109: 345-350.

Roach, R. and Hackett, P. H. (2001). Frontiers of hypoxia research: acute mountain sickness. The Journal of Experimental Biology 204: 3161-3170.

Roach, R. C., Bartsch, P., Hackett, P. H. and Olez, O. (1993). The Lake Louise Acute Mountain Sickness Scoring System. *In: Hypoxia and Mountain Medicine*. J. R. Sutton, C. S. Houston and G. Coates. Burlington, VT, Queen City Press: 272-274.

Roach, R. C., Greene, E. R., Schoene, R. B. and Hackett, P. H. (1998). Arterial oxygen saturation for prediction of acute mountain sickness. Aviation Space & Environmental Medicine 69(12): 1182-5.

Rodriguez, F. A., Ventura, J. L., Casas, M., Casas, H., Pages, T., Rama, R., Ricart, A., Palacios, L. and Viscor, G. (2000). Erythropoietin acute reaction and haematological adaptations to short, intermittent hypobaric hypoxia. European Journal of Applied Physiology. 82(3): 170-7.

Rusko, H. K., Tikkanen, H., Paavolainen, L., Hamalainen, I., Kalliokoski, K. and Puranen, A. (1999). Effect of living in hypoxia and training in normoxia on sea level VO2max and red cell mass. Medicine & Science in Sports & Exercise 31 (Supplement 5): S86.

Saito, S., Nishihara, F., Takazawa, T., Kanai, M., Aso, C., Shiga, T. and Shimada, H. (1999). Exercise-induced cerebral deoxygenation among untrained trekkers at moderate altitudes. Archives of Environmental Health 54(4): 271-277.

Sanchez del Rio, M. and Moskowita, M. A. (1999). High altitude headache. Hypoxia: Into the Next Millenium. R. C. Roach, Wagner, P. D., Hackett, P. H. New York, Kluwer Academic/Plenum Publishers. 474: 145-154.

Schmidt, W. (2002). Effects of intermittent exposure to high altitude on blood volume and erythropoietic activity. High Altitude Medicine & Biology 3(2): 167-176.

Schoene, R. B. (1982). Control of ventilation in climbers to extreme altitude. Journal of Applied Physiology: Respiratory, Environmental & Exercise Physiology 53(4): 886-90.

Schoene, R. B. (1999). The brain at high altitude. Wilderness & Environmental Medicine 10(2): 93-6.

Schoene, R. B., Roach, R. C., Hackett, P. H., Sutton, J. R., Cymerman, A. and Houston, C. S. (1990). Operation Everest II: ventilatory adaptation during gradual decompression to extreme altitude. Medicine & Science in Sports & Exercise 22(6): 804-10.

Segler, C. P. (2001). Prophylaxis of climbers for prevention of embolic accidents. Medical Hypotheses 57(4): 472-475.

Serebrovskaya, T. V. (2002). Intermittent hypoxia research in the former Soviet Union and the Commonwealth of Independent States: History and review of the concept and selected applications. High Altitude Medicine & Biology 3(2): 205-221.

Severinghaus, J. W. (2001). Cerebral circulation at high altitude. High Altitude: An Exploration of Human Adaptation. T. F. Hornbein, Schoene, R. B. New York, Marcel Dekker, Inc. 161: 343-375.

Severinghaus, J. W., Chiodi, H., Eger, E., Brandstater, B. and Hornbein, T. F. (1966). Cerebral blood flow in man at high altitude. Circulation Research 19: 274-282.

Shah, N., Trivedi, N. K., Clack, S. L., Shah, M., Shah, P. P. and Barker, S. (2000). Impact of hypoxemia on the performance of cerebral oximeter in volunteer subjects. Journal of Neurosurgical Anesthesiology 12(3): 201-209.

Singh, I., Khanna, P. K., Lai, M., Roy, S. B. and Subramanyam, C. S. (1969). Acute mountain sickness. New England Journal of Medicine 280(4): 175-184.

Smith, C. A., Bisgard, G. E., Nielsen, A. M., Daristotle, L., Kressin, N. A., Forster, H. V. and Dempsey, J. A. (1986). Carotid bodies are required for ventilatory acclimatization to chronic hypoxia. Journal of Applied Physiology 60(3): 1003-10.

Tansley, J. G., Fatemian, M., Howard, L. S., Poulin, M. J. and Robbins, P. A. (1998). Changes in respiratory control during and after 48 h of isocapnic and poikilocapnic hypoxia in humans. Journal of Applied Physiology 85(6): 2125-34.

Townsend, N. E., Gore, C. J., Hahn, A. G., McKenna, M. J., Aughey, R. J., Clark, S. A., Kinsman, T., Hawley, J. A. and Chow, C. M. (2002). Living high-training low increases hypoxic ventilatory response of well-trained endurance athletes. Journal of Applied Physiology. 93(4): 1498-505.

Ward, M. P., Milledge, J. S. and West, J. B. (2000). High Altitude Medicine and Physiology. London, Arnold.

Weil, J. V. (1986). Ventilatory control at high altitude. Handbook of Physiology. The Respiratory System. Control of Breathing. A. P. Fisherman, N. S.

Cherniack, J. G. Widdicombe and S. R. Geiger. Baltimore, MD, Williams and Wilkins. II: 703-727.

Weil, J. V., Byrne-Quinn, E., Sodal, I. E., Friesen, W. O., Underhill, B., Filley, G. F. and Grover, R. F. (1970). Hypoxic ventilatory drive in normal man. Journal of Clinical Investigation 49(6): 1061-72.

Wilbur, R. L. (2001). Current trends in altitude training. Sports Medicine 31: 249-265.

Yao, F., Levin, S. K., Wu, D., Illner, P., Yu, J., Huang, S. W. and Tseng, C. C. (2001). Maintaining cerebral oxygen saturation during cardiac surgery shortened ICU and hospital stays. Anesthesia and Analgesia 92(4 supplement): SCA86.

CHAPTER 2

VALIDATION OF PULSE OXIMETRY DURING

PROGRESSIVE NORMOBARIC HYPOXIA

UTILIZING A PORTABLE CHAMBER

2.1   INTRODUCTION

The state of oxygenation is crucial in understanding patient health status, the hypoxia associated with high altitude, or the impact of high intensity exercise. Pulse oximetry provides a simple non-invasive method of estimating the percentage of hemoglobin that is saturated with oxygen (SpO_2), and thus is a valuable diagnostic tool in monitoring subjects or patients during desaturation episodes. Technological advances over the past twenty-five years, and the relative ease of operation combined with continuous data output, have made pulse oximetry the minimal standard of care for patient monitoring during anesthesia as well as an essential tool in the practice of emergency medicine (Tremper and Barker, 1989; Sinex, 1999). Furthermore, there is a growing interest to employ pulse oximeters to detect levels of hypoxemia during intensive exercise (Martin et al., 1992; Benoit et al., 1997; Yamaya et al., 2002), and to monitor the hypoxia associated with high altitude (Roach et al., 1998; Hussain et al., 2001).

Recently, endurance athletes and high altitude climbers have gained access to commercially available portable normobaric hypoxic chambers (NHC) which are used to stimulate physiological changes similar to those observed during acclimatization to altitude or experimental acclimation to hypobaric hypoxia via decompression chambers (Powell and Garcia, 2000). In most cases, the intended use of the portable normobaric hypoxic equipment is to enhance athletic performance or pre-acclimatize mountaineers to the rigor of high altitude expeditions. Pulse oximetry has been utilized as a method to monitor oxygen saturation during NHC exposures (Kolb et al., 2001; Townsend et al., 2002). While pulse oximetry has become a generally acceptable method for the detection and quantification of hypoxemia, numerous reports during the past decade have shown that pulse oximeters become inaccurate during desaturation events both at rest (Grace, 1994; Trivedi et al., 1997; Thrush and Hodges, 1994) and during exercise (Wood, et al., 1997; Yamaya et al., 2002). The magnitude of the error depends on the specific monitor, location of sensor, and the degree of hypoxia (Sinex, 1999). Given that NHC are capable of eliciting a wide range of hypoxia (F_IO_2 20.9% to 9.5%), and that at present there are no guidelines describing appropriate level or time-frame of hypoxic exposures, investigations are warranted to address the basic efficacy of the altitude simulation chambers and the validation of pulse oximeters employed to monitor human subjects. However, to our knowledge, there are no scientific studies which have tested the reliability of pulse oximetry measurements against recognized standards in response to the hypoxia generated by commercially available NHC. The general aim of the present investigation was to compare non-invasive pulse oximetry with direct arterial blood measurements via co-oximetry throughout the condition of progressive normobaric hypoxia. The specific aims of this study were to address three main questions. Firstly, is SpO_2 a valid estimate of SaO_2 at the levels of normobaric hypoxia typically used in research and recreational settings?

Secondly, is there any affect of the location of pulse oximetry sensors in estimating SpO_2? Finally, are changes in SpO_2 and SaO_2 similar relative to the severity of hypoxemia?

2.2   METHODS

2.2.1   Subjects

Thirteen subjects (6 women, 7 men) aged 21.3 ± 0.6 years (mean$\pm$SD) volunteered to participate in the study. All subjects were healthy non-smokers, and were not taking any medication. None reported any history of cardiovascular, cerebrovascular, or respiratory disease. Each volunteer gave informed consent according to ethical guidelines approved for this study by the Conjoint Health Research Ethics Board, University of Calgary.

2.2.2   Experimental Design

The project utilized a modified one-group time series design (Campbell and Stanley, 1966) that incorporated sequential single-subject analyses during the treatment protocol, in order to compare two methods, which measure the same factor (Altman and Bland, 1983). The method of co-oximetry provided direct arterial blood measurements of SaO_2 for comparison against non-invasive pulse oximetry estimates of oxy-hemoglobin saturation. Method comparisons were made from a total of seven arterial blood samples, collected from each subject at designated intervals, during the progressive normobaric hypoxic exposure (procedure described below).

2.2.3 Progressive Normobaric Hypoxia

A NHC equipped with air separation generators (Hypoxico, Inc., New York, NY, USA), was used to progressively reduce the normoxic F_IO_2 of 20.9% over a 150 min period to an endpoint F_IO_2 of approximately 11.5%. The choice of hypoxic exposure is well supported in the literature for both normobaric and hypobaric investigations (Benoit et al., 1992; Rodriguez et al., 1999), while the time frame provided ideal logistical conditions for blood sampling and analysis. The F_IO_2 inside the NHC was monitored on a continuous basis throughout the progressive normobaric hypoxic exposure using a TrueMax 2400 Metabolic Measurement System (ParvoMedics; Salt Lake City, USA).

2.2.4 Pulse Oximetry

HR and SpO_2 were continuously monitored via pulse oximetry (Nellcor N-295, Nellcor Inc. Hayward, Ca, USA). The non-invasive computerized monitor, with memory storage and capable of real-time download, was attached to the subject's index finger using a comfortable near infrared light emitting diode (LED) probe (D-25) secured in place with opaque tape to prevent signal artifacts from fluorescent lighting. Additionally, a second set of pulse oximetry data was obtained from each subject, via a separate monitor with an LED probe (RS-10) placed over the eyebrow relative to the pulsatile events of the anterior branch of the temporal artery. The dual sets of probes were established to retrieve information regarding possible variability of SpO_2 measurements between the sites (site dependency).

2.2.5   Blood Samples and Analyses

Radial artery catheterization was established and monitored by a physician. Prior to entering the hypoxic room an initial 1 ml of blood was drawn into a sterile, heparinized syringe under ambient atmospheric conditions (inspired fraction of oxygen (F_IO_2) = 20.9%). The second sample was obtained following 15 min of hypoxic exposure. The remaining five blood collections occurred at 30 min intervals while the F_IO_2 was progressively reduced to approximately 11.5%. Blood gas analysis and co-oximetry measurements were performed immediately following sample collection. Arterial blood samples were assessed for pH, $PaCO_2$, PaO_2, HCO_3, base excess, and total hemoglobin concentration, with a CIBA-CORNING 280 Blood Gas Analyser (East Walpole, MA, USA). The blood gas analyzer is equipped with a pre-heater which warmed each blood sample to 37°C prior to entering the electrode sample path. Non-hemolyzing co-oximetry assays of oxyhemoglobin fraction (FO_2Hb), carboxyhemoglobin fraction (FCOHb), methemoglobin fraction (FMETHb) and total hemoglobin were acquired with a AVOXimeter 4000 (San Antonio TX, USA). Strong precision and accuracy (oxy-hemoglobin linear relationship, $R^2 = 0.999$, precision = 0.85%, bias = 0.04%) of the AVOXimeter 4000 compared with a conventional IL 482 co-oximeter has been previously reported (Bailey et al., 1997). To obtain SaO_2, or functional saturation, for direct comparison with pulse oximetry SpO_2 data, the following equation (AVOX Systems, 2001) was employed:

$$SaO_2 = 100 \text{ x } FO_2Hb / 100 - (FCOHb + FM_{ET}Hb)$$

Both the CIBA-CORNING Blood Gas Analyzer and the AVOXimeter 4000 were calibrated daily using standard procedures according to the manufacturer's specifications.

2.2.6   Synchronization of Blood Measurements with Pulse Oximetry

The internal digital timing mechanisms for each pulse oximeter (one with a temporal probe and the other with a finger probe) were synchronized exactly to within 1 sec. The Nellcor NPB-295 stored HR and SpO_2 data at two-second intervals throughout the experimental treatment. An event marker was recorded to identify the precise moment that each blood sample was drawn. The F_IO_2 inside the chamber was also recorded during each blood sampling procedure. Subsequently, a 40 sec interval of pulse oximetry data (20 sec on either side of the blood collection event), was used for comparison with the direct blood gas analysis.

2.2.7   Statistical Analysis

The correlation between the direct blood measurements of SaO_2 and the non-invasive indirect measurements from the two pulse oximetry devices (SpO_2) were initially evaluated using parametric statistics. Pearson product moment correlation coefficients, R^2, and regression analyses were examined between the dependent variables. To examine differences between regression lines, the Chow Test (Dillon and Goldstein, 1984) was utilized to assess whether the coefficients estimated over one group of the data were equal to the coefficients estimated over another group of data. Significance was accepted at $P < 0.05$. To further address the accuracy of the difference between the instruments, method comparison analysis was utilized (Altman and Bland, 1983; Bland and Altman, 1986). First, the differences between the methods of measurement for each collection period were determined (n=84). Then the bias (b), or the mean value between the differences of SaO_2 and SpO_2, in conjunction with precision (p), or the standard deviation of the differences, were calculated to graphically illustrate the limits of agreement between the methods. These lines of identity then represent the 95% confidence interval, or ±2 standard deviations of the differences:

$$b = SaO_2 - SpO_2 / n\text{-}1$$

$$p = SD \text{ of } (SaO_2 - SpO_2) = SD_{diff}$$

$$Limits \text{ of Agreement} = b \pm 2SD_{diff}$$

2.3   RESULTS

2.3.1   General

Summary data obtained from co-oximetry, blood gas analysis, and pulse oximetry
for all subjects during the progressive normobaric hypoxia is illustrated in Figure
1. The summary graph, constructed from the means of all data points (n=84)
during each of the synchronized blood collection events, illustrates decreasing
SaO_2 and SpO_2 throughout the progressive hypoxic protocol (lower panel). The
upper panel of Figure 1 illustrates an initial rapid decline in PaO_2 (partial pressure
of arterial oxygen), which continued at a slower rate of descent from
approximately 65 mmHg to 40 mmHg as the normobaric hypoxia progressed
from an F_iO_2 of approximately 20% to 11.5%. In contrast, the $PaCO_2$ (partial
pressure of arterial carbon dioxide) demonstrated a small decrease over the period
of hypoxia.

2.3.2   Linear Regressions and the Chow Test

Regression analysis between SaO_2 measured from direct blood samples and SpO_2
estimated with pulse oximetry are presented in Figure 2 (all observations) and
Figure 3 (observations < 85%). Both $SpO_{2temporal}$ (LED probe RS-10) and $SpO_{2finger}$
(LED probe D-25) were highly correlated with co-oximetry SaO_2 (R^2 = 0.92 and
0.89 respectively). However, the strength of the correlation between co-oximetry
and both pulse oximetry devices (temporal and finger) was substantially reduced
when blood saturation levels below 85% were compared (n=26). When co-

Figure 2.1

Mean data obtained from all observations (n = 84) for co-oximetry and pulse oximetry (lower panel), and arterial blood gases (upper panel) during the progressive normobaric hypoxia. SpO_2 finger data was obtained with the D-25 sensor, while the RS-10 sensor was employed for SpO_2 temporal data collection. Symbols: □ = PaO_2 (mmHg), ■ = $PaCO_2$ (mmHg), ● with solid line = SaO_2 (%), ▲ with short dash line = SpO_2 finger (%), ◇ with long dash line = SpO_2 temporal (%). Values are Mean ± SD.

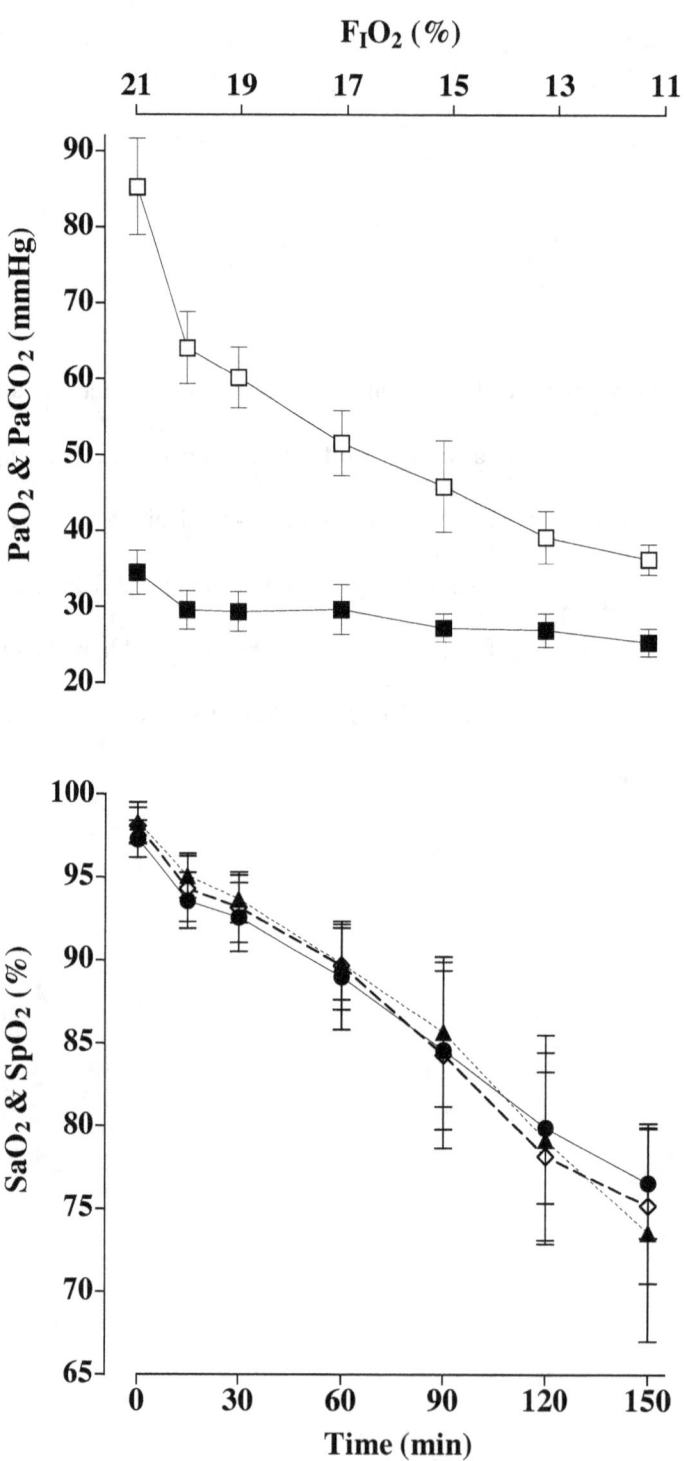

Figure 2.2

Regression lines (Left), and limits of agreement (Right) for all data points (n = 84) comparing SpO_2 temporal (RS-10) (Panels A and C) and SpO_2 finger (D-25) (Panels B and D) with SaO_2. Long and thick dash lines represent ± 95% confidence interval; short and thin dash line identifies the bias. Values for limits of agreement and regression analysis are presented in Table 1.

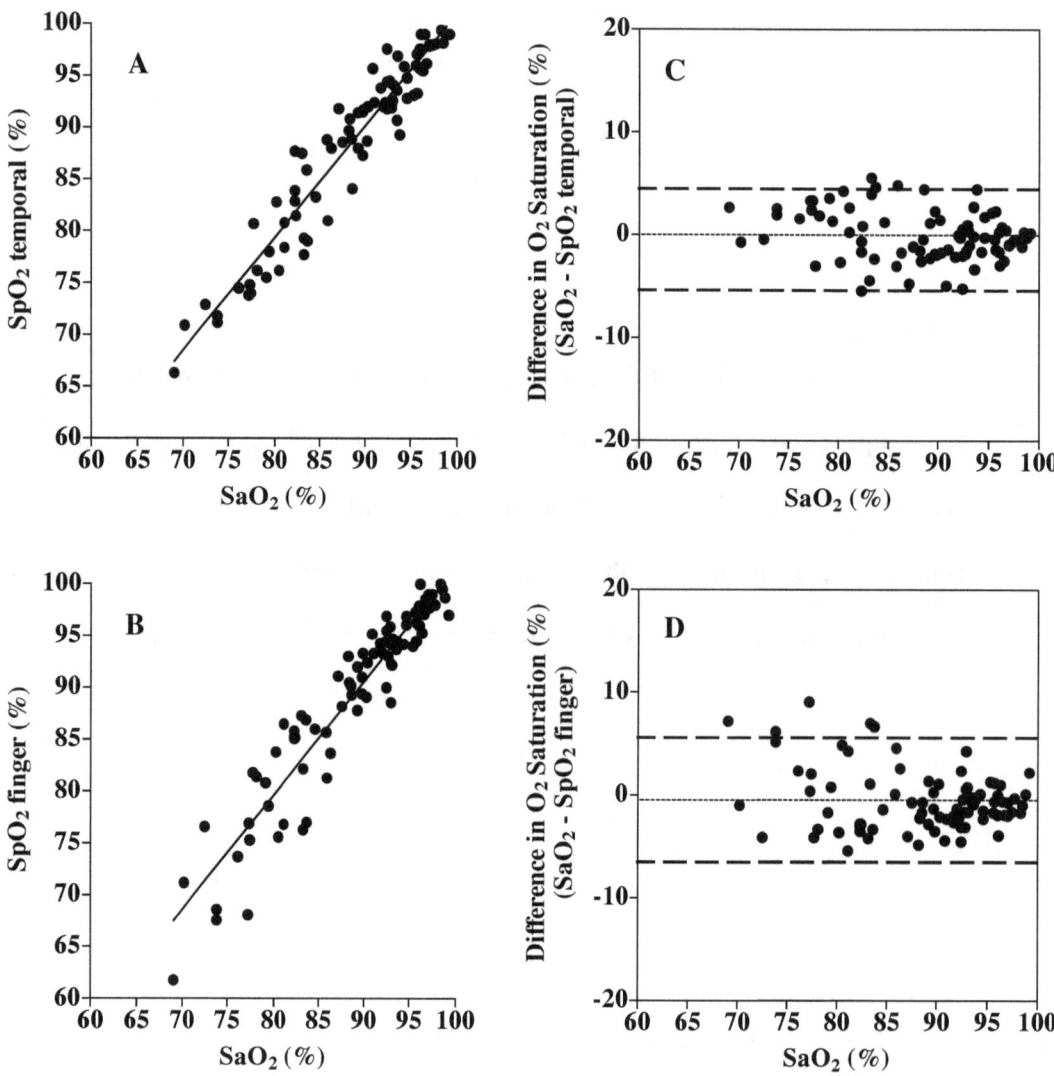

Figure 2.3

Regression lines (Left), and limits of agreement (Right) for all SaO_2 < 85%

observations (n = 26) comparing SpO_2 temporal (RS-10) (Panels A and C) and

SpO_2 finger (D-25) (Panels B and D) with SaO_2. Long and thick dash lines

represent ± 95% confidence interval; short and thin dash line identifies the bias.

Values for limits of agreement and regression analysis are presented in Table 1.

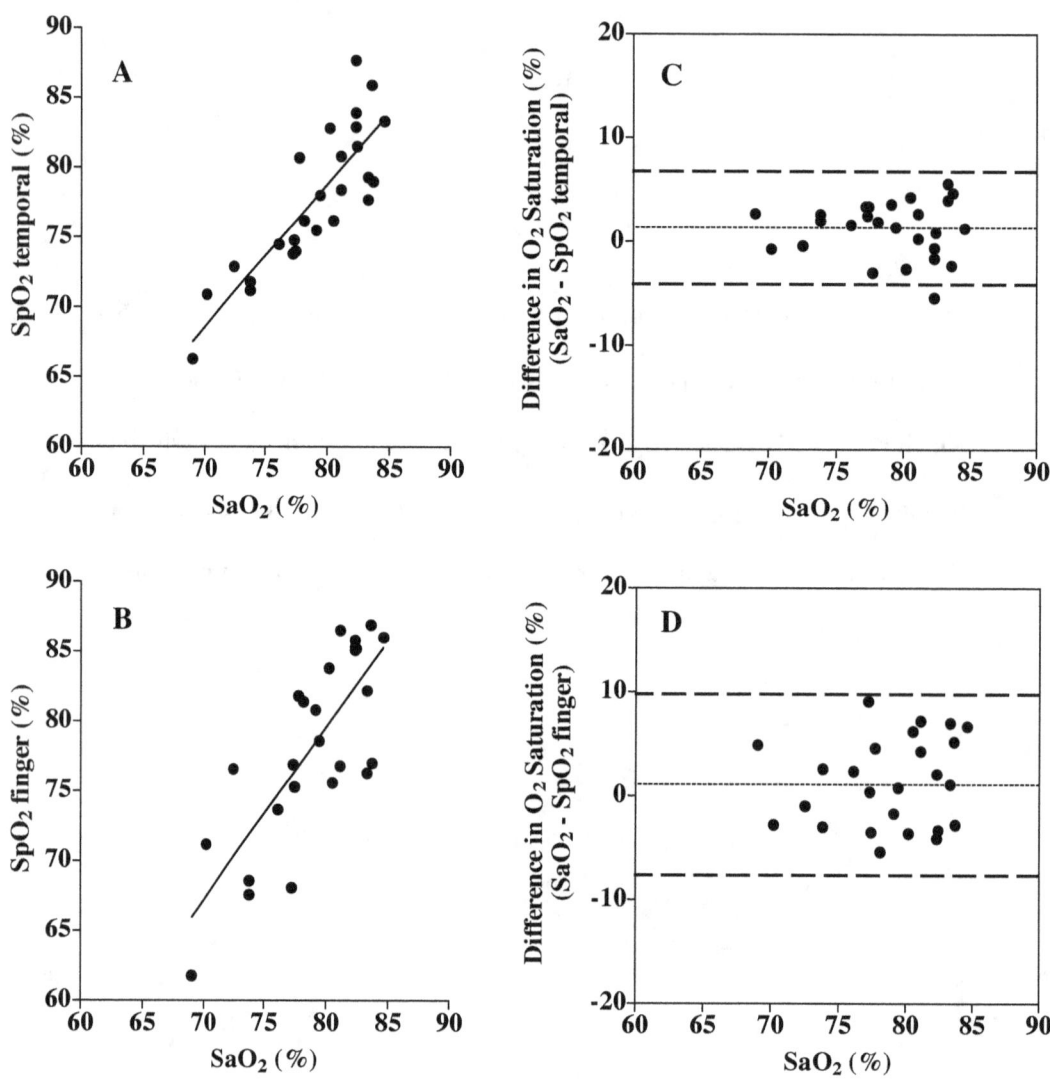

oximetry $SaO_2 < 85\%$ was compared with SpO_2, the temporal probe had a much higher R^2 relative to the finger probe ($R^2 = 0.71$ and 0.56 respectively). The Chow Test identified significant differences occurred between the methods when all of the data from $SpO_{2temporal}$ and $SpO_{2finger}$ was compared with $SpO_{2finger} < 85\%$ ($P < 0.001$).

2.3.3 Assessment of Agreement Between Methods of Measurement

The results for b and p between SaO_2 and $SpO_{2temporal}$ and $SpO_{2finger}$ are presented in Figure 2 (all observations) and Figure 3 (observations $< 85\%$) adjacent to regression lines. Relative to site specificity of the two LED probes when averaging all of the data, the RS-10 temporal probe had the lowest b and greatest p compared to the D-25 finger probe (b, p = 0.016, 2.47 versus 0.47, 3.03 respectively). The b for $SpO_2 < 85\%$ was similar for both LED probes while p was much greater for the temporal probe in comparison to the finger probe (1.37, 2.72 versus 1.12, 4.34 respectively). Summary for the limits of agreement and regression analysis is presented in Table 1.

Table 2.1

Method comparison data showing regression correlation and limits of agreement.

Methods	R^2	Slope	Intercept	Bias	Precision	95% CI
SaO_2 vs $SpO_{2temporal}$	0.92	1.08	-7.33	0.02	2.47	-5.41 to 4.47
SaO_2 vs $SpO_{2finger}$	0.89	1.10	-8.56	-0.47	3.03	-6.52 to 5.58
SaO_2 vs $SpO_{2temporal}$ < 85%	0.73	1.02	-2.80	1.38	2.72	-4.06 to 6.82
SaO_2 vs $SpO_{2finger}$ < 85%	0.56	1.19	-15.90	1.13	4.34	-7.55 to 9.81

Abbreviations and Definitions: $SpO_{2temporal}$ = arterial oxygen saturation via pulse oximeter with probe placed over the anterior branch of the temporal artery (RS-10), $SpO_{2finger}$ = arterial oxygen saturation via pulse oximeter with probe placed on the index finger (D-25), < 85% = incorporates hypoxic data points below 85%. (CI = confidence interval).

2.4   DISCUSSION

There are three new findings that emerge from this study. First, pulse oximeters provide reasonable accuracy for estimating arterial oxygen saturation in a NHC when $SaO_2 > 85\%$. However, the accuracy of the oximetry devices used in this experiment deteriorated as hypoxemia increased.   Second, in response to progressive normobaric hypoxia the RS-10 (temporal probe) provided greater validity than did the D-25 (finger probe) when compared to *in vitro* arterial blood samples analyzed by co-oximetry. The enhanced performance of the temporal probe is reflected by a higher correlation, smaller *b*, greater *p*, and a narrower ± 95% confidence interval in the study sample from this investigation.   Third, when the data was limited to low saturation levels ($< 85\%$), the finger probe performed significantly inferior when compared against the temporal probe ($P < 0.001$).

2.4.1   Site Dependency

Given that the pulse oximetry monitors used in this investigation operated with identical algorithms for estimating SpO_2, the discrepancy between the temporal probe (RS-10) and finger probe (D-25) may have likely been due to specific site location and / or design differences between the probes. The temporal probe is a 'reflectance' instrument with the LED and detector on the same side of the tissue, while the finger probe is a ' transmission' instrument that emits light through the fingernail, tissue, and blood with a detecting sensor located on the opposite side of the digit. In the present investigation, the finger probe was placed on the right index finger as per the manufacturers directions while the temporal probe site was identified by palpation of the anterior branch of the temporal artery above the eyebrow, followed by a brief search for the area which generated the highest arterial saturation and strongest plethysmography event.

Some controversy exists in the literature relative to the effect which pulsating arteries have on reflectance pulse oximetry probes in that a number of authors have reported enhanced performance (Dassel et al., 1995; Trivedi et al., 1997), while others suggest deterioration in accuracy (Kelleher and Ruff, 1989; Jorgensen et al., 1995; Hamber et al., 1999). Reduced accuracy of reflectance pulse oximetry has been reported in endotracheally intubated and ventilated adults undergoing general anesthesia and surgery, as well as in adult volunteers placed in the Trendelenberg (head–down tilt) position (Jorgensen et al., 1995). Of note is a contrary report that advocates a small amount of pressure (7.3 to 11.9 kPa) applied to reflectance probes located on the forehead, improves SpO_2 accuracy (Dassel et al., 1995). Interestingly, the RS-10 temporal probe used in the present investigation, was held in place with an elastic headband, which exerted some pressure on the sensor against the skin of the forehead that may have augmented performance.

Seven pulse oximeters (reflectance and transmission) were examined for accuracy and response time (sensitivity) to a single brief (30-90 sec) hypoxic event (F_iO_2 =

10%) engendered via reduced oxygen gas mixtures (Trivedi et al., 1997). While all devices exhibited varying levels of inaccuracy at low saturations (b range = 1.2 to 8.5, p range = ± 3.1 to 7.5), the Nellcor 200 reflectance probe, placed on the forehead, and the Ohmeda ear probe exhibited the best performance. Trivedi and collegues (1997) suggested that the reflectance forehead probe and ear probe may have monitored desaturation events more accurately and faster due to their placement being 'central' as opposed to the 'peripheral' finger probe location. It is possible that the issue of central vs. peripheral site dependency may have contributed to the improved performance of the 'centrally' fixed Nellcor RS-10 temporal probe reported in the present findings. In support of this, centrally located ear probes have been recently identified to produce significantly ($P <$ 0.05) enhanced performance during desaturations of $SaO_2 < 90\%$ when compared with probes which were located peripherally on the finger and toe (Hamber et al., 1999).

Similar pulse oximetry devices to those utilized during our NHC protocol at rest were evaluated by Yamaya et al. (2002) in response to exercise while breathing hypoxic gas (F_IO_2 = 12%). Our results for the RS-10 temporal probe (b = 0.02, p = 2.47) compare favorably with those of Yamaya and colleagues (b = 0.3, p = 2.5). However our findings suggest that the performance of the D-25 finger probe is more accurate during rest (b = -0.47, p = 3.03) than during hypoxic exercise (b = -1.4, b = 7.9). Factors responsible for the discrepancy between rest and exercise may be associated with exercise induced peripheral vasoconstriction causing reduced perfusion at the site of measurement, or the motion artifact induced by exercise (Severinghaus and Kelleher, 1992). Collectively, our results and those reported by Yamaya et al. (2002), suggest that during hypoxic episodes, both at rest and during exercise, reflectance pulse oximetry probes are more reliable than transmission probes.

2.4.2   Low Levels of Oxygen Saturation

Yelderman et al. (Yelderman and William, 1983) compared direct arterial blood oxygen saturation with results from a pulse oximeter fitted with a finger probe. Seventy-nine data points were obtained from five subjects exposed to stepwise hypoxia to SaO_2 of approximately 70%. They reported a correlation coefficient of 0.98. Examination of their scatter plot, however, suggests that variability may have increased at lower saturations. Furthermore, they did not present data regarding b (mean differences) or p (standard deviation of the differences). Despite strong correlations between pulse oximetry and SaO_2, care should be expressed in the interpretation of the data presented by Yelderman et al. since strong bivariate relationships do not necessarily imply agreement between the two methods (Atkinson and Nevill, 2000). Alternatively, a rapid desaturation technique utilizing compressed low oxygen delivered by a mouth piece, assessed the accuracy of 14 pulse oximeters whilst addressing the agreement between methods (Severinghaus et al., 1989). Seven probes were of the finger type while the remaining seven were reflectance forehead probes. When compared to co-oximetry SaO_2, the correlation coefficients for these devices ranged from $R^2 = 0.81$ to 0.96. At very low saturations of approximately 55%, the average b varied greatly (-21.60 to 1.86) while average p also demonstrated considerable variability (2.46 to 9.26).

More recently, the accuracy of four pulse oximeters were examined using healthy adults at rest in response to hypoxic stages of $SaO_2 < 80\%$, $85 - 90\%$, $90 - 95\%$, and $95 - 100\%$ (Thrush and Hodges, 1994). They reported a statistically significant ($P < 0.05$) deterioration in accuracy from all four devices as oxygen saturation decreased. Concern of the reliability of pulse oximetry was expressed by Thrush and Hodges (1994) when they revealed numerous falsely elevated SpO_2 values above 90% when SaO_2 measurements (co-oximetry) for the same subjects were below 90%, suggesting that greater degrees of hypoxemia were elicited than was indicated by the pulse oximeters. When saturations below 80% were analyzed using method comparisons, b varied from 0 to 2 while p ranged from ±3 to 5. Our findings for both temporal RS–10 and finger D–25 probes for oxygen saturation levels < 85% are consistent with the data of Thrush and Hodges (1994).

2.4.3   Conclusion

In summary, the pulse oximetry devices used in the present investigation operated with higher accuracy and precision, under the condition of progressive normobaric hypoxia established with air separation generators, when the arterial oxygen saturation was > 85%. Thus, SpO_2 is a valid estimate of SaO_2 when SaO_2 > 85%.   In the sample population from this study, reflectance sensor probes obtained significantly better pulse oximetry recordings than did transmission probes when SaO_2 was < 85%, suggesting that design differences or that location (central vs. peripheral) may impact performance during low levels of oxygen saturation. From a practical perspective, results from this study suggest that pulse oximetry provides reliable monitoring of hypoxemia at rest when utilizing normobaric hypoxic chambers within the range of 20.9% to 15% F_iO_2; equivalent to an altitude range of between sea level and approximately 3500m (Ward et al., 2000).   Practical relevance for exercise is beyond the scope of this paper. However, some useful information can be derived from studies at rest. It is important to recognize that all pulse oximeters estimate *in vivo* arterial oxygen saturation by measuring the light absorbance of hemoglobin at two different wavelengths, and additionally that there are numerous differences in the algorithms and filtering methods used by individual manufacturers to determine SpO_2. In this regard, caution should be taken when monitoring individuals with pulse oximetry, especially those exposed to low saturation levels generated by normobaric hypoxia. It would appear prudent, that when regular use of commercially available normobaric hypoxic chambers is expected, the pulse oximetry devices used to assess SpO_2 should be validated against arterial blood measurements to ensure the health status of the user.

2.5   REFERENCES

Altman, D. G. and Bland, J. M. (1983). The analysis of method comparison studies. The Statistician 32: 307-317.

Atkinson, G. and Nevill, A. (2000). Typical error versus limits of agreement. Sports Medeicine 30(375-381): 375-381.

AVOX Systems (2001). AVOXimeter 4000 Operator's & Service Manual: 61.

Bailey, S. R., Russel, E. L. and Martinez, A. (1997). Evaluation of the Avoximeter: Precision, long-term stability, linearity, and use without heparin. Journal of Clinical Monitoring 13: 191-198.

Benoit, H., Costes, F., Feasson, L., Lacour, J. R., Roche, F., Denis, C., Geyssant, A. and Barthelemy, J. C. (1997). Accuracy of pulse oximetry during intense exercise under severe hypoxic conditions. European Journal of Applied Physiology 76(3): 260-263.

Benoit, H., Germain, M., Barthelemy, J. C., Denis, C., Castells, J., Dormois, D., Lacour, J. R. and Geyssant, A. (1992). Pre-acclimatization to high altitude using exercise with normobaric hypoxic gas mixtures. International Journal of Sports Medicine 13(Suppl 1): S213-6.

Bland, J. M. and Altman, D. G. (1986). Statistical methods for assessing agreement between two methods of clinical measurement. Lancet 1(8476): 307-10.

Campbell, D. T. and Stanley, J. C. (1966). Experimental and Quasi-experimental Designs for Research. Chicago, Rand McNally and Company.

Dassel, A. C., Graaff, R., Sikkema, M., Meijer, A., Zijlstra, W. G. and Aarnoudse, J. G. (1995). Reflectance pulse oximetry at the forehead improves by pressure on the probe. Journal of Clinical Monitoring 11: 237-244.

Dillon, W. R. and Goldstein, M. (1984). Multivariate Analysis: Methods and Applications. New York, John Wiley and Sons Inc.

Grace, R. F. (1994). Pulse oximetry. Gold standard or false sense of security? Medical Journal of Australia 160:638-644.

Hamber, E. A., Bailey, P. L., James, S. W., Wells, D. T., Lu, J. K. and Pace, N. L. (1999). Delays in the detection of hypoxemia due to site of pulse oximetry probe placement. Journal of Clinical Anesthesia 11(2): 113-118.

Hussain, M. M., Aslam, M. and Khan, Z. (2001). Acute mountain sickness score and hypoxemia. Journal of the Pakistan Medical Association 51(5): 173-179.

Jorgensen, J., Schmid, E. R., Konig, V., Faisst, K., Huch, A. and Huch, R. (1995). Limitations of forhead pulse oximetry. Journal of Clinical Monitoring 11: 253-256.

Kelleher, J. F. and Ruff, R. H. (1989). The penumbra effect: Vasomotion-dependent pulse oximeter artifact due to probe malposition. Anesthesiology 71: 787-791.

Kolb, J., Norris, S., Smith, D., Henderson, J. and Hillis, F. (2001). Intermittent normobaric hypoxia enhances acclimation. High Altitude Medicine and Biology 2(1): 109.

Martin, D., Powers, S., Cicale, M., Collop, N., Huang, D. and Criswell, D. (1992). Validity of pulse oximetry during exercise in elite endurance athletes. Journal of Applied Physiology 72(2): 455-458.

Powell, F. and Garcia, N. (2000). Physiological effects of intermittent hypoxia. High Altitude Medicine and Biology 1(2): 125-136.

Roach, R. C., Greene, E. R., Schoene, R. B. and Hackett, P. H. (1998). Arterial oxygen saturation for prediction of acute mountain sickness. Aviation Space and Environmental Medicine 69(12): 1182-5.

Rodriguez, F. A., Casas, H., Casas, M., Pages, T., Rama, R., Ricart, A., Ventura, J. L., Ibanez, J. and Viscor, G. (1999). Intermittent hypobaric hypoxia stimulates erythropoiesis and improves aerobic capacity. Medicine and Science in Sports and Exercise 31(2): 264-8.

Severinghaus, J. W. and Kelleher, J. F. (1992). Recent developments in pulse oximetry. Anesthesiology 76:1018-1038.

Severinghaus, J. W., Naifeh, K. and Koh, S. (1989). Errors during profound hypoxia in 14 pulse oximeters. Journal of Clinical Monitoring 5: 72-81.

Sinex, J. E. (1999). Pulse oximetry: Principles and limitations. American Journal of Emergency Medicine 17(1): 59-66.

Thrush, D. and Hodges, M. R. (1994). Accuracy of pulse oximetry during hypoxemia. Southern Medical Journal 87(4): 518-521.

Townsend, N., Gore, C., Hahn, A., McKenna, M., Aughey, R., Clark, S., Kinsman, T., Hawley, J. and Chow, C. (2002). Living high-training low increases hypoxic ventilatory response of well-trained endurance athletes. Journal of Applied Physiology 93: 149-1505.

Tremper, K. K. and Barker, S. J. (1989). Pulse oximetry. Anesthesiology 70(1): 98-108.

Trivedi, N. S., Ghouri, A. F., Lai, E., Shah, N. K. and Barker, S. J. (1997). Pulse oximeter performance during desaturation and resaturation: A comparison of seven models. Journal of Clinical Anesthesia 9(3): 184-188.

Ward, P. M., Milledge, J. S. and West, J.B. (2000). High Altitude Medicine and Physiology. 3rd Ed. London, Arnold.

Wood, R. J., Gore, C. J., Hahn, A. G., Norton, K. I., Scroop, G. C., Campbell, D. P., Watson, D. B., and Emonson, D. L. (1997). Accuracy of two pulse oximeters during maximal cycling exercise. Australian Journal of Science and Medicine in Sport 29:47-50.

Yamaya, Y., Bogaard, H. J., Wagner, P. D., Niizeki, K. and Hopkins, S. R. (2002). Validity of pulse oximetry during maximal exercise in normoxia, hypoxia, and hyperoxia. Journal of Applied Physiology 92: 162-168.

Yelderman, M. and William, N., Jr. (1983). Evaluation of pulse oximetry. Anesthesiology 59: 349-352.

CHAPTER 3

PROTOCOL FOR DETERMINING THE ACUTE

CEREBROVASCULAR AND VENTILATORY

RESPONSES TO ISOCAPNIC HYPOXIA IN HUMANS

3.1   INTRODUCTION

During the past fifty years, numerous studies have been carried out to describe the changes in ventilation, cerebral blood flow (CBF), or cerebral oxygenation that occur during the process of acclimatization to the hypoxia of altitude. Such studies have helped elucidate the potential role that changes in ventilatory and cerebrovascular control may have on the etiology of diseases such as acute mountain sickness, high altitude cerebral edema and high altitude pulmonary edema.

However, to our knowledge no study has yet described the *simultaneous* changes in the acute ventilatory and cerebrovascular responses to hypoxia within the same protocol on the same subjects. To be effective, such a protocol should consist of several levels of hypoxia, and the period spent at each level of hypoxia must be sufficiently long for both the ventilatory and CBF responses to unfold, but short enough to prevent the development of hypoxic ventilatory decline (HVD).

In 1976, Severinghaus suggested that 2 minutes was a suitable time period for the full ventilatory response to hypoxia to develop (Severinghaus, 1976). Conversely, in 1994 Howard and Robbins reported that a protocol consisting of 2-min at seven levels of hypoxia did not result in ventilations which were independent of the order of the hypoxic exposures. In other words, their results showed a significant degree of HVD. More recently, a study was published in this journal, which described a protocol that consisted of 50-sec at seven levels of hypoxia, which resulted in ventilatory responses that were independent of whether the order of the hypoxic exposures increased or decreased; these results suggested the absence of HVD (Mou et al., 1995). However, whilst the protocol of Mou et al. (1995) is adequate to allow the acute ventilatory responses to develop, it is probably not optimal for the measurement of CBF because the duration of each hypoxic step is likely too short for the CBF transients to unfold and for the measurements of CBF to take place (Poulin and Robbins, 1996).

The purpose of this study was to extend the protocol of Mou et al. (1995) by developing a protocol that is suitable for assessing the form of *both* the acute ventilatory and cerebrovascular responses to hypoxia. Such a protocol should be sufficiently long for the cerebrovascular response to develop, but short enough to prevent HVD from occurring.

3.2 METHODS

Thirteen healthy, non-smoking adult males (26.7 ± 3.6 (SD) yrs) volunteered for this study, which was approved by the Conjoint Health Research Ethics Board, University of Calgary. All subjects visited the laboratory (1103m above sea level, average barometric pressure for the study days was 668 ± 11 Torr) on three occasions. During the initial visit, measurements of resting end-tidal P_{O_2} ($P_{ET_{O_2}}$) and P_{CO_2} ($P_{ET_{CO_2}}$) along with estimates of hypoxic and hypercapnic sensitivities were conducted, and the subjects became familiarized with the apparatus and experimental testing procedures. The experimental tests were conducted on the second (*Day 1*) and third (*Day 5*) visits, which were separated by five days. Subjects reported to the laboratory at the same time each morning following an overnight fast. On each of these visits, the subject's normal $P_{ET_{O_2}}$ and $P_{ET_{CO_2}}$ values were measured prior to the experiment, while the subject was sitting quietly and comfortably for approximately 10 min. The respired gases were sampled via a fine catheter held at the opening of one nostril by an adapted nasal O_2 therapy kit. The gas was sampled continuously at a rate of 20 ml/min and analyzed for P_{O_2} and P_{CO_2} by mass spectrometer (AMIS 2000, Innovision, Odense, Denmark). Values for P_{O_2} and P_{CO_2} were sampled by computer every 10 ms. The values for $P_{ET_{O_2}}$ and $P_{ET_{CO_2}}$ were determined and recorded for each breath using a computer and dedicated software (Chamber v1.00, University Laboratory of Physiology, Oxford, UK).

3.2.1   Incremental Hypoxic and Hypercapnic Protocol

The experimental protocol began with an eight-minute period during which the subject breathed normally through a mouthpiece with the nose occluded by a nose clip.   Respiratory volumes and flow information were obtained with a pneumotachograph and differential pressure transducer (RSS100-HR, Hans Rudolf Inc., Kansas City, MO, USA).   Respiratory flow direction and timing information were measured with a turbine volume transducer (VMM-400, Interface Associates, CA, USA).   Accurate control of the end-tidal gases was achieved using the technique of dynamic end-tidal forcing (BreatheM v2.07, University Laboratory of Physiology, Oxford, UK).   A controlling computer generated the inspired partial pressure of O_2 and CO_2 predicted to give the desired end-tidal partial pressures by using a fast gas mixing system (Robbins et al., 1982; Howson et al., 1987; Ide et al., 2003).   The controlling computer received feedback of the measured end-tidal partial pressures on a breath-by-breath basis as the experiment progressed.   These measured end-tidal values were then compared with the desired values, and the computer adjusted the initial predicted inspired gas mixture by using an integral proportional feedback algorithm based on the deviations of the measured end-tidal values from the desired end-tidal values (Robbins et al., 1982).

After an eight minute lead-in period consisting of eucapnic euoxia ($P_{ET_{O_2}}$ = 88

Torr) the hypoxic stimulus was altered by holding the P_{ETO_2} at 7 different predetermined levels over the range of 88-45 Torr while the P_{ETCO_2} was held constant at eucapnia (1.5 Torr above the subject's resting value). These levels were calculated to provide equal steps in oxygen saturation of the arterial blood, by using the relationship described by Severinghaus (1979). Eucapnic euoxia was followed by descending steps of hypoxia (P_{ETO_2} = 75.2, 64.0, 57.0, 52.0, 48.2, and 45.0 Torr), each step lasting 90 sec (Fig 1). Immediately after the last hypoxic step, an additional 10-min period was incorporated into the protocol to provide a simple measurement of acute hypercapnic sensitivity. For this part of the protocol, P_{ETO_2} was elevated to 300 Torr for 5 min while P_{ETCO_2} remained at eucapnia. Then, P_{ETCO_2} was raised an additional 7.5 Torr for 5 min whilst P_{ETO_2} remained constant at 300 Torr. The final ten minutes of this protocol served to establish the changes in the acute ventilatory and cerebrovascular responses to hypercapnia. Arterial oxygen saturation (SpO_2) was measured continuously throughout each experiment via pulse oximetry (3900 Pulse Oximeter, Datex-Ohmeda, Mississauga, Canada).

Figure 3.1

Schematic of the experimental protocol illustrating the desired time-related

alterations of end-tidal PO_2 ($P_{ET_{O_2}}$), arterial oxygen saturation (SaO_2), and end-

tidal PCO_2 ($P_{ET_{CO_2}}$).

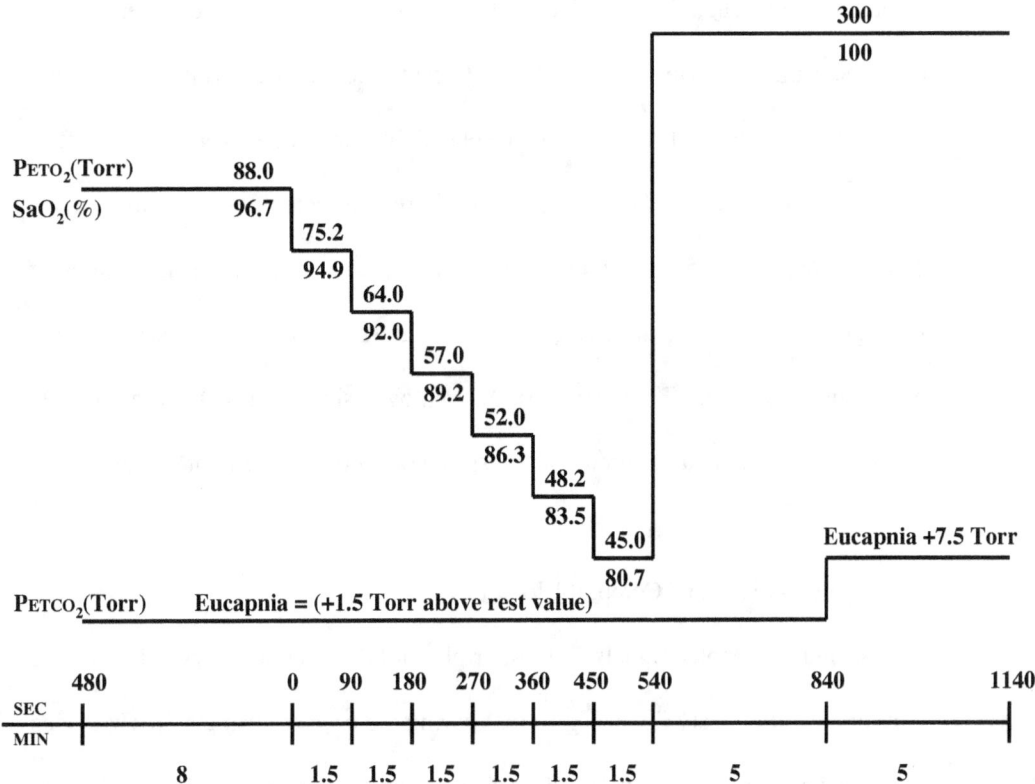

3.2.2   Measurement of Cerebral Oxygenation

Throughout the protocol, near-infrared spectroscopy was used to monitor regional cerebral oxygen saturation (S_tO_2) in the brain (INVOS 4100, TYCO Health Care Group Canada Inc., Pointe-Claire, QC, Canada).   A light emitting diode (SomaSensor, Tyco Health Care Group Canada Inc.) was carefully placed over the right front-temporal region of the forehead, just above the eyebrow and left of the midsaggital sulcus.   The SomaSensor alternately generates two wavelengths of light (730 and 805nm) which detect oxygenated and deoxygenated states of hemoglobin to estimate an index of oxygen saturation based on internal micro-processing algorithms (Kim et al., 2000). Analogue signals of S_tO_2 were obtained every 2 sec throughout the protocol and stored on a computer for later analysis.

3.2.3   Measurement of Cerebral Blood Flow

Backscattered Doppler signals from the right middle cerebral artery (MCA) were measured continuously (ie. every 10 ms) during the protocol using a 2MHz pulsed Doppler Ultrasound system (TC22, SciMed, Bristol, England).   The MCA was identified by an insonation pathway through the right temporal window just above the zygomatic arch by using search techniques described previously (Poulin and Robbins, 1996). The Doppler probe was secured with a headband device (Müller and Moll Fixation, Nicolet Instruments, Madison, Wisconsin, USA) to maintain optimal insonation position and angle throughout the protocol. In this study, the peak blood velocity (VP) was acquired every 10 ms and averaged over each heart beat ($\overline{\text{V}}_\text{P}$), and this was used as the primary index of CBF   (Poulin and Robbins, 1996).

3.2.4   Analysis

The acute hypoxic ventilatory response (AHVR), the acute hypoxic cerebral blood flow response (AHR$_\text{CBF}$), and the acute hypoxic cerebral oxygenation response (AHRS$_\text{r}$O$_2$) were determined by linear regression between the mean ventilation ($\dot{\text{V}}_\text{E}$), $\overline{\text{V}}_\text{P}$, S$_\text{r}O_2$ and arterial oxygen saturation (100-SaO$_2$) during the final 20 sec of each incremental step of hypoxia.   The acute ventilatory response to hypercapnia (AHCVR), the acute hypercapnic cerebral blood flow response (AHCR$_\text{CBF}$) and the acute hypercapnic cerebral oxygenation response (AHCRS$_\text{r}$O$_2$) were determined by linear regression between the mean $\dot{\text{V}}_\text{E}$, $\overline{\text{V}}_\text{P}$, S$_\text{r}O_2$ and P$_\text{ET}$CO$_2$ during the final two minutes of the hyperoxic-eucapnic and hyperoxic-hypercapnic steps.   The variability in the cerebrovascular and ventilatory responses between *Day 1* and *Day 5* were assessed by determining the coefficients of variation ((standard deviation of the difference / grand mean) x 100).   Furthermore, the cerebrovascular and ventilatory responses to hypoxia and hypercapnia between *Day 1* and *Day 5* were compared statistically using a student paired t-test.

3.3   RESULTS

All subjects tolerated the hypoxic protocol well. Results of a typical experimental protocol in one subject (ID# 0053) are shown in Fig 2. This figure illustrates that the $P_{ET}CO_2$ was well controlled throughout the experimental protocol. Fig 3. illustrates the mean values across all subjects for $P_{ET}CO_2$ (top panel) throughout the seven levels of hypoxia. The three lower panels of Fig 3. illustrate the ventilatory response ($\dot{V}E$), CBF response ($\overline{V}_P$), and cerebral oxygenation response (S_rO_2) to hypoxia.

Individual subject means for *Day 1* and *Day 5* for the measurements of AHVR, AHCVR, AHR$_{CBF}$, AHCR$_{CBF}$, AHRs$_rO_2$, and AHCRs$_rO_2$ are summarized in Table 1. The average coefficients of variation between *Day 1* and *Day 5* were 15.2% (AHVR), 7.9% (AHCVR), 10.4% (AHR$_{CBF}$), 2.9% (AHCR$_{CBF}$), 8.0% (AHRs$_rO_2$), and 3.9% (AHCRs$_rO_2$). Within-group means for CBF, ventilatory, and S_rO_2 sensitivity to hypoxia and hypercapnia on *Day 1* and *Day 5* are presented in Fig 4. Paired t-tests of the sensitivities between *Day 1* and *Day 5* revealed no significant differences illustrating that the cerebrovascular and ventilatory sensitivities to hypoxia and hypercapnia were similar on the two separate experimental days.

Figure 3.2

Sample experimental protocol for one subject (ID# 0053). $\overline{V}_P$, middle cerebral artery peak blood velocity; S_rO_2, regional cerebral oxygen saturation; SpO_2, arterial oxygen saturation (pulse oximetry); $\dot{V}_E$, ventilation; $P_{ET_{O_2}}$, end-tidal PO_2 (solid line); $P_{ET_{CO_2}}$, end-tidal PCO_2 (dashed line). Each data point represents an average over 20 s.

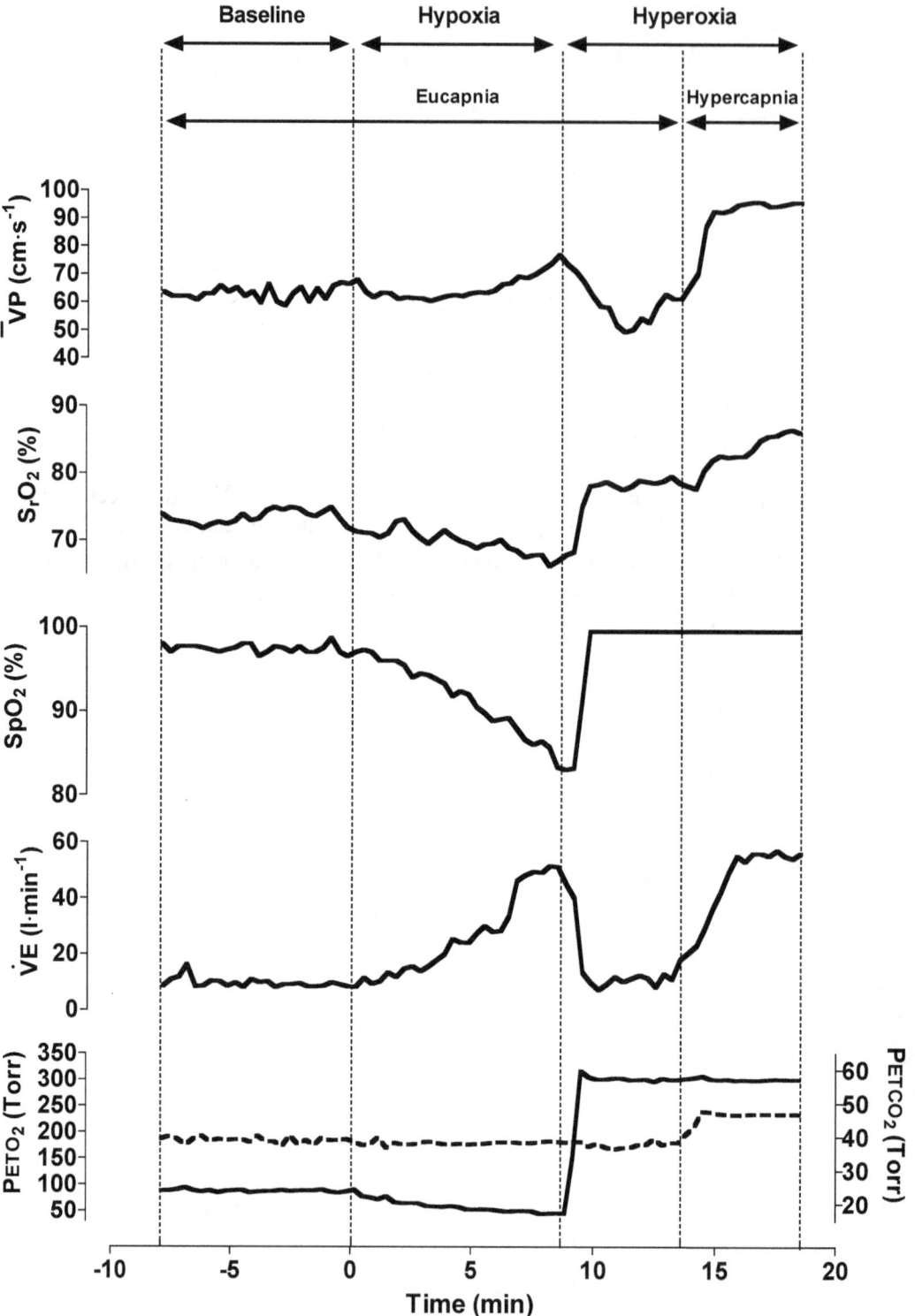

Table 3.1
Mean values from the experimental protocol for each subject.

Subject No.	AHVR (l·min^{-1}·%$^{-1}$)	AHCVR (l·min^{-1}·Torr^{-1})	AHR$_{CBF}$ (cm·s^{-1}·%$^{-1}$)	AHCR$_{CBF}$ (cm·s^{-1}·Torr^{-1})	AHRS$_r$O$_2$ (%·%$^{-1}$)	AHCRS$_r$O$_2$ (%·Torr^{-1})
0004	0.62±0.04	2.51±0.24	0.48±0.06	2.01±0.36	0.56±0.14	1.22±0.13
0005	0.90±0.05	2.54±0.30	0.58±0.16	1.88±0.07	0.99±0.12	1.10±0.05
0044	1.49±0.00	4.51±0.31	0.36±0.12	1.86±0.82	0.89±0.02	0.71±0.09
0048	0.66±0.13	4.88±1.73	0.32±0.12	1.76±1.56	0.58±0.11	1.21±0.01
0049	0.77±0.59	3.99±0.18	0.37±0.23	2.97±1.13	0.89±0.10	1.12±0.07
0051	1.70±0.27	1.73±0.07	0.57±0.13	2.42±0.32	0.87±0.06	0.92±0.14
0052	1.64±0.74	3.40±1.00	0.53±0.08	3.50±1.06	0.73±0.20	1.16±0.08
0053	2.20±0.13	4.01±0.90	0.44±0.05	1.90±0.48	0.74±0.08	0.80±0.11
0054	0.60±0.24	1.49±1.14	0.40±0.22	2.61±0.12	0.72±0.17	1.04±0.11
0057	3.60±0.53	8.93±0.64	0.86±0.17	3.56±1.22	0.85±0.06	1.15±0.00
0058	0.74±0.17	2.71±0.55	0.26±0.06	2.42±0.21	0.88±0.11	0.90±0.01
0059	0.68±0.28	1.65±0.33	0.28±0.08	1.87±0.06	0.78±0.01	1.16±0.16
0060	0.47±0.11	1.60±0.34	0.27±0.00	1.70±0.12	0.90±0.02	1.22±0.09
Mean	1.24±0.89	3.38±2.03	0.43±0.18	2.34±0.65	0.80±0.13	1.05±0.17
CV, %	15.2	7.9	10.4	2.9	8.0	3.9

Individual subject values are means±SD for *Day 1* and *Day 5*. AHVR, acute hypoxic ventilatory response; AHCVR, acute hypercapnic ventilatory response; AHR$_{CBF}$, acute hypoxic cerebral blood flow response; AHCR$_{CBF}$, acute hypercapnic cerebral blood flow response; AHRS$_r$O$_2$, acute hypoxic cerebral oxygenation response; AHCRS$_r$O$_2$, acute hypercapnic cerebral oxygenation response; CV, coefficient of variation.

Figure 3.3

Relationship between $P_{ET_{O_2}}$ and $\dot{V}_E$, $\overline{V}_P$, S_rO_2, and $P_{ET_{CO_2}}$ during the eucapnic

hypoxia protocol, averaged across all subjects. Error bars are ± 1 S.E.M.

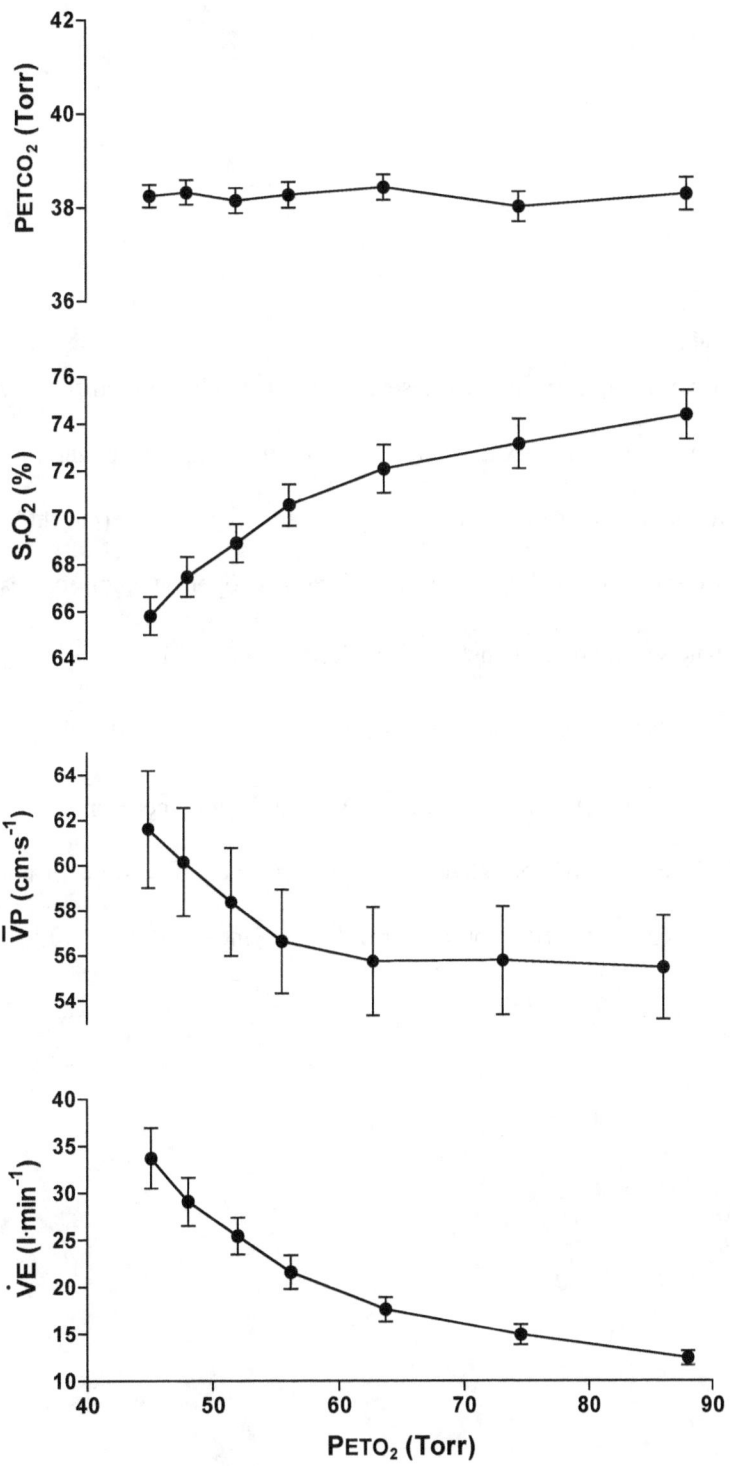

Figure 3.4

Between day measurements of the sensitivity of cerebral blood flow ($\dot{V}$ P) and

ventilation ($\dot{V}$E) to hypoxia (panel A) and hypercapnia (panel B) and the

sensitivity of cerebral oxygenation to hypoxia and hypercapnia (panel C). Closed

symbols correspond to hypoxic sensitivities and open symbols correspond to

hypercapnic sensitivities. Panel A: ● = slope of $\dot{V}$E and 100-SaO$_2$, ▲ = slope of

$\overline{V}$P and 100-SaO $_2$ in response to the incremental step changes of isocapnic

hypoxia. Panel B: ○ and △ = slopes of $\dot{V}$E and $\overline{V}$P to hypercapnia, respectively.

Panel C: ■ = slope of normalized S$_r$O$_2$ and 100-SaO$_2$ □ = slope of normalized

S$_r$O$_2$ response to CO$_2$,. Symbols and error bars are means ± SD (n = 13 subjects).

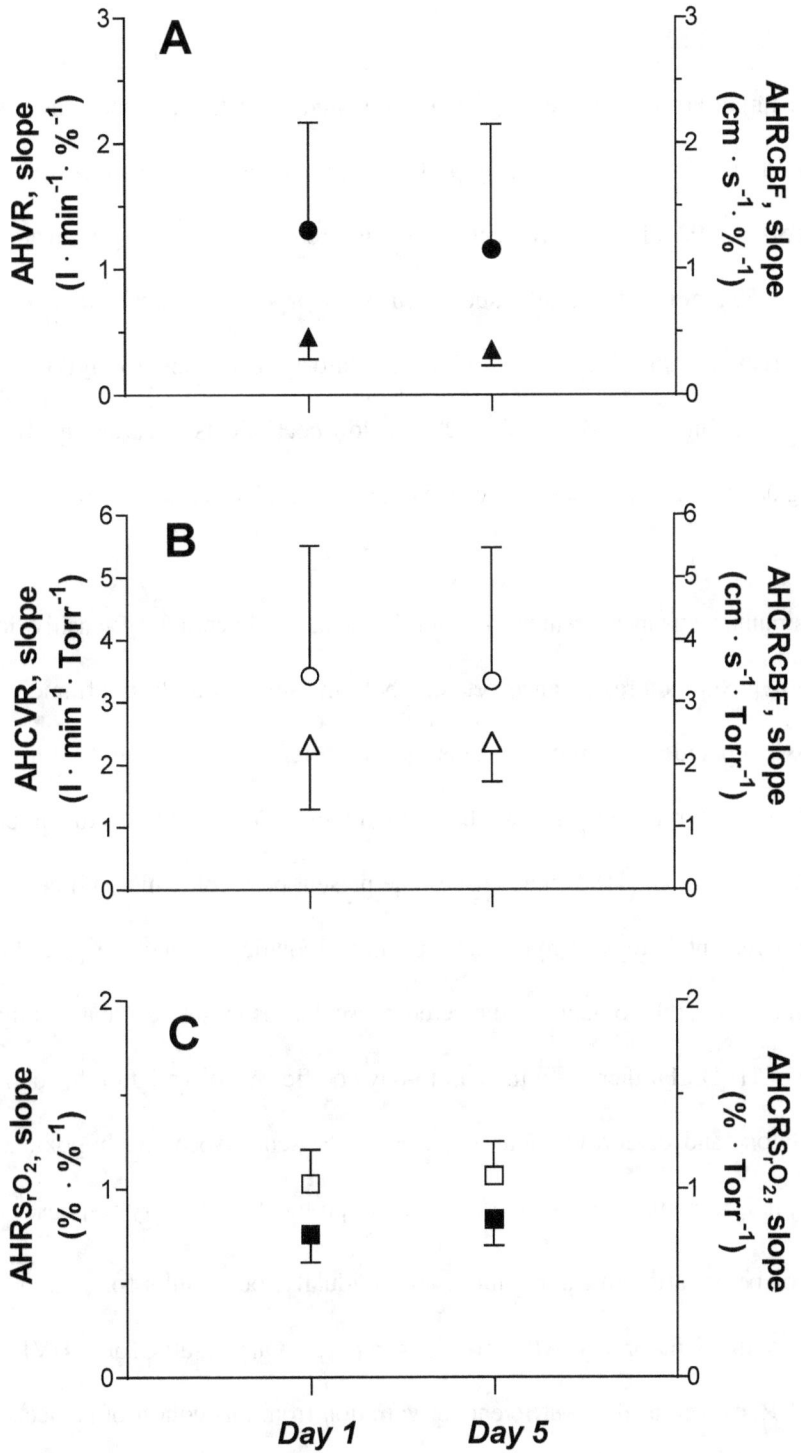

3.4   DISCUSSION

Three important findings emerge from this study. First, we extend the results reported by Mou et al. (1995), by prolonging the duration of each hypoxic step from 50 s to 90 s in an incremental hypoxic protocol without any indication of HVD. Secondly, this study successfully incorporates both CBF and S_rO_2 measurements simultaneously with ventilatory responses to hypoxia and hypercapnia into one protocol. Thirdly, the low coefficients of variation advocate strong day-to-day reproducibility of the outcome variables in this protocol.

The simultaneous measurement of cerebrovascular and ventilatory sensitivities to acute hypoxia requires balance between both the severity and time frame of the hypoxic episode. If the stimulus is too brief, both the ventilatory and cerebrovascular responses may be incomplete. Conversely, if the hypoxic stimulus is too long, HVD may ensue. The present protocol, which utilizes seven 90 s incremental steps of hypoxia, appears to provide an adequate period over which it is possible to quantify the cerebrovascular responses, while avoiding the onset of HVD. Furthermore, the day-to-day coefficients of variation for both the ventilatory and cerebrovascular sensitivities to acute isocapnic hypoxia were small, indicating the feasibility of the present protocol to quantify responses over time or before/after an intervention. Individually, our results for $\dot{V}_E$, $\overline{V}_P$ and S_rO_2 compare favorably with previous reports. Our results for AHVR and AHCVR, as well as the coefficients of variation from this cohort of subjects, are comparable with those reported by others (Zhang and Robbins 1995). The $\overline{V}_P$ responses to hypoxia and hypercapnia are also comparable with previous reports (Poulin et al., 2002), while the S_rO_2 response compares favorably with cerebral oxygenation changes to variations of hypoxia and CO_2 reported by Imray et al. (2000). Collectively, our results show the feasibility of incorporating measurements of $\dot{V}_E$, $\overline{V}_P$ and S_rO_2 within one protocol to yield estimates of acute sensitivities to hypoxia and hypercapnia.

3.4.1 Practical Considerations and Summary

The process of acclimatization to the hypoxia of altitude is associated with changes in ventilation (Basu et al., 1996; Tansley et al., 1998) and cerebral blood flow (Jensen et al., 1996; Severinghaus, 2001; Poulin et al., 2002). However, the role of changes in CBF on the ventilatory acclimatization to hypoxia (VAH) and in the etiology of acute mountain sickness (AMS) and high altitude cerebral edema (HACE) remains unclear (Roach and Hackett, 2001). The ventilatory sensitivity to hypoxia is highly variable between subjects, and a blunted chemosensitivity to hypoxia has been reported to contribute to the susceptibility of AMS via a reduction in SaO_2 (Moore et al., 1986; Matsuzawa et al., 1989; Ricart et al., 2000). Furthermore, in the first reported investigation monitoring S_rO_2 at various altitudes (2270, 3650, and 4680m) AMS symptomatology worsened as cerebral oxygenation declined ($r = -0.41$, $P < 0.05$) (Imray et al., 1998). Subsequently, cerebral oxygen desaturation has been observed in unacclimatized trekkers to an altitude of 4300m (Saito et al., 1999). In their study, Saito et al. (1999) suggested that the acute reduction in S_rO_2, followed by an increase in CBF, might be a primary cause of headache and AMS.

In summary, this protocol appears well suited to quantify the cerebrovascular and ventilatory responses to acute isocapnic hypoxia. Moreover, it may help further elucidate the role of changes in CBF in VAH with chronic or intermittent hypoxia, or in the etiology of diseases such as AMS and HACE.

3.5 REFERENCES

Basu, C. K., Selvamurthy, W., Bhaumick, G., Gautam, R. K. and Sawhney, R. C. (1996). Respiratory changes during initial days of acclimatization to increasing altitudes. Aviation Space and Environmental Medicine 67: 40-5.

Howard, L. S. and Robbins, P. A. (1994). Problems with determining the hypoxic response in humans using stepwise changes in end-tidal PO_2. Respiration Physiology 98: 241-9.

Howson, M. G., Khamnei, S., McIntyre, M. E., O'Connor, D. F. and Robbins, P. A. (1987). A rapid computer controlled binary gas mixing system for studies in respiratory control. Journal of Physiology 394: 7P.

Ide, K., Eliasziw, M. and Poulin, M. J. (2003). The relationship between middle cerebral artery blood velocity and end-tidal PCO_2 in the hypocapnic-hypercapnic range in humans. Journal of Applied Physiology 95: 129-137.

Imray, C. H. E., Barnett, N. J., Walsh, S., Clarke, T., Morgan, J., Hale, D., Hoar, H., Mole, D., Chesner, I. and Wright, A. D. (1998). Near-infrared spectroscopy in the assessment of cerebral oxygenation at high altitude. Wilderness and Environmental Medicine 9: 198-203.

Imray, C. H. E., Brearey, S., Clarke, T., Hale, D., Morgan, J., Walsh, S. and Wright, A. D. (2000). Cerebral oxygenation at high altitude and the response to carbon dioxide, hyperventilation and oxygen. Clinical Science 98: 159-164.

Jensen, J. B., Sperling, B., Severinghaus, J. W. and Lassen, N. A. (1996). Augmented hypoxic cerebral vasodilation in men during 5 days at 3,810 m altitude. Journal of Applied Physiology 80: 1214-8.

Kim, M. B., Ward, D. S., Cartwright, C. R., Kolano, J., Chelhowski, S. and Henson, L. C. (2000). Estimation of jugular venous O_2 saturation from cerebral oximetry or arterial O_2 saturation during isocapnic hypoxia. Journal of Clinical Monitoring 16: 191-199.

Matsuzawa, Y., Fujimoto, K., Kobayashi, T., Namushi, N. R., Harada, K., Kohno, H., Fukushima, M. and Kusama, S. (1989). Blunted hypoxic ventilatory drive in subjects susceptible to high-altitude pulmonary edema. Journal of Applied Physiology 66: 1152-7.

Moore, L. G., Harrison, G. L., McCullough, R. E., McCullough, R. G., Micco, A. J., Tucker, A., Weil, J. V. and Reeves, J. T. (1986). Low acute hypoxic ventilatory response and hypoxic depression in acute altitude sickness. Journal of Applied Physiology 60: 1407-12.

Mou, X. B., Howard, L. S. and Robbins, P. A. (1995). A protocol for determining the shape of the ventilatory response to hypoxia in humans. Respiration Physiology 101: 139-43.

Poulin, M. J., Fatemian, M., Tansley, J. G., O'Connor, D. F. and Robbins, P. A. (2002). Changes in cerebral blood flow during and after 48 h of both isocapnic and poikilocapnic hypoxia in humans. Experimental Physiology 87.5: 633-642.

Poulin, M. J. and Robbins, P. A. (1996). Indexes of flow and cross-sectional area of the middle cerebral artery using Doppler ultrasound during hypoxia and hypercapnia in humans. Stroke 27: 2244-2250.

Ricart, A., Casas, H., Casas, M., Pages, T., Palacios, L., Rama, R., Rodriguez, F. A., Viscor, G. and Ventura, J. L. (2000). Acclimatization near home? Early respiratory changes after short-term intermittent exposure to simulated altitude. Wilderness and Environmental Medicine 11: 84-8.

Roach, R. C. and Hackett, P. H. (2001). Frontiers of hypoxia research: acute mountain sickness. Journal of Experimental Biology 204: 3161-3170.

Robbins, P. A., Swanson, G. D. and Howson, M. G. (1982). A prediction correction scheme for forcing alveolar gases along certain time courses. Journal of Applied Physiology 52: 1353-1357.

Saito, S., Nishihara, F., Takazawa, T., Kanai, M., Aso, C., Shiga, T. and Shimada, H. (1999). Exercise-induced cerebral deoxygenation among untrained trekkers at moderate altitudes. Archives of Environvironmental Health 54: 271-277.

Severinghaus, J. W. (1976). Proposed standard determination of ventilatory responses to hypoxia and hypercapnia in man. Chest 70: 129-131.

Severinghaus, J. W. (1979). Simple, accurate equations for human blood O_2 dissociation computations. Journal of Applied Physiology 46: 599-602.

Severinghaus, J. W. (2001). Cerebral circulation at high altitude. In: Horbein, T.F., Schoene, R.B. (Eds). Lung Biology in Health and Disease, Vol. 161: High Altitude: An Exploration of Human Adaptation. Marcel Dekker, Inc., New York, pp. 343-375

Tansley, J. G., Fatemian, M., Howard, L. S., Poulin, M. J. and Robbins, P. A. (1998). Changes in respiratory control during and after 48 h of isocapnic and poikilocapnic hypoxia in humans. Journal of Applied Physiology 85: 2125-34.

Zhang, S. and Robbins, P. A. (2000). Methodological and physiological variability within the ventilatory response to hypoxia in humans. Journal of Applied Physiology 88: 1924-32.

CHAPTER 4

EFFECTS OF 5 CONSECUTIVE NOCTURNAL HYPOXIC EXPOSURES ON THE VENTILATORY RESPONSES TO ACUTE HYPOXIA AND HYPERCAPNIA IN HUMANS

4.1 INTRODUCTION

Alterations in respiratory control during periods of either chronic or intermittent hypoxic exposures seem to be facilitated by two main processes, which contribute to the increase in ventilation and a reciprocal decrease in end-tidal P_{CO_2} ($P_{ET CO_2}$). The first of these processes is an increase in the acute hypoxic ventilatory response (AHVR). An increase in the AHVR allows ventilatory acclimatization to altitude to proceed, despite respiratory alkalosis and a withdrawal of the stimulus to the chemoreceptors (Dempsey and Forster, 1982). The second process is evident in a leftward shift of the acute hypercapnic ventilatory response (AHCVR), and also in an increase in the slope of this relationship, which is normally determined under euoxic or hyperoxic conditions. The leftward shift in the AHCVR has been suggested to be related to the degree of re-setting of the central chemoreceptors to start responding to a lowered P_{CO_2} (Cunningham et al., 1986).

Several studies have demonstrated a progressive increase in the AHVR during both natural altitude acclimatization (Forster et al., 1971; Reeves et al., 1993; Sato et al., 1994) and intermittent hypoxic exposures (Levine et al. 1992; Katayama et al., 1998; Garcia et al., 2000; Mahamed and Duffin, 2001; Townsend et al., 2002). During natural altitude acclimatization, a leftward shift of the AHCVR has been well documented (Hasselbalch and Lindhard, 1911; Kellogg et al., 1957; Forster et al., 1971; White et al., 1987; Schoene et al., 1990). However, the effect of intermittent exposure to hypoxia on AHCVR has received little investigation. In one study, subjects were exposed to a simulated altitude of 4,500m for 6 consecutive days (30 min·day^{-1}) (Katayama et al., 1998). Whilst there was a significant increase in AHVR, there were no reported differences in the AHCVR (Katayama et al., 1998). This lack of change in the AHCVR is perhaps not surprising, due to the brevity of exposure, since such changes would likely require marked decreases in $P_{ET_{CO_2}}$ and subsequent respiratory alkalosis to elicit changes at the site of the central chemoreceptors.

In contrast, some studies employing a modified rebreathing technique have provided data to suggest that the enhancement of the AHVR following 14 days of intermittent hypoxia (20 min·day^{-1}) was produced by a decrease in the threshold of the peripheral chemoreflex ventilatory response to carbon dioxide, rather than an increase in sensitivity (Mahamed and Duffin, 2001). The authors interpreted this decrease in threshold as indicating an increase in the overall activity of the peripheral chemoreflex for any giving level of stimulus. The same group showed similar results following 3 hours of isocapnic hypoxia (Mahamed et al., 2003). However, during both these investigations, neither baseline ventilation nor $P_{ET_{CO_2}}$ was different following the hypoxic interventions (Mahamed and Duffin, 2001; Mahamed et al., 2003).

The general aim of the present study was to generate an intermittent hypoxic exposure, which would elicit marked decreases in $P_{ET_{CO_2}}$ and subsequent respiratory alkalosis. To achieve this, twelve male subjects slept 8-9 $h \cdot day^{-1}$ overnight for 5 consecutive days at a simulated attitude of 4300 m. The specific aim of this study was to address three main questions. First, is the magnitude of the AHVR similar to that previously reported in other intermittent and chronic hypoxic studies? Second, would 5 nights of hypoxia, at a simulated attitude of 4,300 m, elicit a change in the slope and/or intercept of the AHCVR? Finally, is the time frame of ventilatory acclimatization and de-acclimatization similar? We tested the specific hypothesis that 5 consecutive nights of normobaric hypoxia would elicit similar changes in respiratory control to those reported during chronic altitude exposures.

4.2   METHODS

4.2.1   Subjects

Twelve healthy male subjects (26.6 ± 4.1 (SD) yrs) participated in this study. All subjects were given both verbal and written instructions outlining the experimental procedure, and written informed consent was obtained. Participants were not taking any medication, all were non-smokers, and none had any history of cardiovascular, cerebrovascular, or respiratory disease. The research study was approved by the Conjoint Health Research Ethics Board at the University of Calgary.

4.2.2   Protocol

The experiments were conducted in a laboratory located at 1103 m above sea level, and the average barometric pressure for the study days was 667 ± 14 Torr. One week prior to the study, each subject was required to make three visits to the laboratory. During the initial visit, measurements of resting end-tidal gases and estimates of hypoxic and hypercapnic sensitivities were conducted, and the subjects became familiarized with the apparatus and experimental testing procedures.

For all subsequent testing, subjects reported to the laboratory at the same time of day following an overnight fast. The control measurements were conducted on the second and third visits. Both control measurements were separated by 5 days.

Following the final control measurement, each subject underwent 5 consecutive nights of normobaric hypoxia at a simulated altitude of ~4,300 m (FiO_2 = ~13.8%: PiO_2 = ~85 Torr). Subjects entered the tents (Hypoxico, Inc) by approximately 22:00 hrs and left at 07:00 hrs the following morning. In between the hypoxic exposures, subjects maintained their normal daily activities. Following the third night of hypoxic exposure, the subjects reported back to the laboratory for another baseline arterialized blood sample (described in section 2.4). After the 5 nights of intermittent hypoxia subjects were permitted to go home but were asked to maintain their normal diet and physical activity levels.

Immediately following the 5 nights of hypoxic exposures, and after 5 days of recovery, subjects reported to the laboratory to repeat the control tests. On each of these visits, the subjects normal PET_{CO_2} and end-tidal O_2 tension (PET_{O_2}) was measured prior to the experiment, while the subject was sitting quietly and comfortably for approximately 10 min. The respired gas was sampled via a fine catheter held at the opening of one nostril by an adapted nasal O_2 therapy kit. The gas was sampled continuously at a rate of 20 ml/min and analyzed for P_{O_2} and P_{CO_2} by mass spectrometer (AMIS 2000, Innovision, Odense, Denmark). Values for P_{O_2} and P_{CO_2} were sampled by a computer every 10 ms. PET_{O_2} and PET_{CO_2} were identified and recorded for each breath using a computer and dedicated software (Chamber v1.00, University Laboratory of Physiology, Oxford, UK). Following the 10 min of resting data, the subjects' AHVR, ventilation in hyperoxia ($\dot{V}E$ hyperoxia) and AHCVR were then assessed, as described in section 2.3 below.

4.2.3 Measurements of AHVR, $\dot{V}E$ hyperoxia and AHCVR

Measurements of AHVR and $\dot{V}E$ hyperoxia were conducted at all times with the PET_{CO_2} held at 1.5 mmHg above the subjects initial air-breathing value before the start of the hypoxic exposures. As mentioned, prior to the 5 nights of hypoxic exposure, the subjects' resting PET_{O_2} and PET_{CO_2} was measured during the initial visit and then again during the 2 control tests prior to the AHVR, $\dot{V}E$ hyperoxia and AHCVR tests. During both the control tests, the between-day coefficients of variation for measurement of PET_{CO_2}, AHVR, $\dot{V}E$ hyperoxia and AHCVR were 5.5%, 17%, 14%, and 7.9%, respectively.

4.2.3.1 AHVR
Following an initial eight-minute lead in period of eucapnic euoxia (PET_{O_2} = 88 Torr), the hypoxic stimulus to the peripheral chemoreceptors was varied by holding the PET_{O_2} at 6 descending steps (PET_{O_2} = 75.2, 64.0, 57.0, 52.0, 48.2, and 45.0 Torr), each step lasting 90 sec. The PET_{CO_2} was held constant 1.5 Torr above resting during the hypoxic challenge. These levels were calculated to provide equal steps in oxygen saturation of the arterial blood, and consequently a linear increase in ventilation over time, via the relationship described by Severinghaus

(1977). A linear regression was then performed between the mean values for ventilation and 100 - SaO_2 during the final 20 sec of each step. The slope of this relationship yielded numerical values for AHVR; this represents an index of the sensitivity to hypoxia (Mou et al., 1995).

4.2.3.2 $\dot{V}E$ hyperoxia and AHCVR

Immediately following the measurement of AHVR, the PET_{O_2} was elevated to 300 Torr for 5 min while PET_{CO_2} remained at eucapnia. The last 2 min of this period was averaged and used to determine $\dot{V}E$ hyperoxia. Then, $P_{ET_{CO_2}}$ was raised rapidly over 1-2 breaths by an additional 7.5 Torr for 5 min whilst PET_{O_2} remained constant at 300 Torr. Combined with the results from the measurements of $\dot{V}E$ hyperoxia, the last 2 min of the hypercapnic period was used to calculate the AHCVR.

Additionally, in 2 subjects who completed the hypoxic exposure, we conducted the AHVR and AHCVR tests at a PET_{CO_2} level that should have produced the same arterial pH as that occurred during the control tests. The matched arterial pH- PET_{CO_2} level was calculated using the relationship described by Michel et al. (1966) from the pH, P_{CO_2}, Hb content, and saturation of the arterialized blood samples. This method of conducting respiratory control tests at a matched arterial pH has been described previously (Tansley et al., 1998) as a method to account for any significant changes in acid-base balance through renal compensation or from other process from the hypoxic exposures.

During the tests, the technique of dynamic end-tidal forcing was used to control $P_{ET_{CO_2}}$ and $P_{ET_{O_2}}$. In brief, the inspired and expired gases were sampled at a rate of 20 ml/min and analyzed by mass spectrometer for fractional concentrations of O_2 and CO_2. Respiratory volumes and flow information were obtained by using a pneumotachograph and differential pressure transducer (RSS100-HR, Hans Rudolph Inc., Kansas City, MO, USA). Respiratory flow direction and timing information were measured with a turbine volume transducer (VMM-400, Interface Associates, CA, USA). A computer sampled the experimental variables every 10 ms. Accurate control of the end-tidal gases was achieved using the technique of dynamic end-tidal forcing (BreatheM v2.07, University Laboratory of Physiology, Oxford, UK). A controlling computer generated the inspired partial pressure of O_2 and CO_2 predicted to give the desired end-tidal partial pressures by using a fast gas mixing system (Robbins et al., 1982; Howson et al., 1987; Ide et al., 2003). The controlling computer received feedback of the measured end-tidal partial pressures on a breath-by-breath basis as the experiment progressed. These measured end-tidal values were compared with the desired values, and the computer then adjusted the initial predicted inspired gas mixture by using an integral proportional feedback algorithm based on the deviations of

the measured end-tidal values from the desired end-tidal values (Robbins et al.,
1982).

4.2.4   Blood Sampling

Capillary blood samples from the ear lobe were taken shortly after arriving to the
laboratory, after 10-15 min of rest. In an attempt to arterialize the blood sample,
topical analgesic cream (Zostrix, Medcis, Quebec, Canada) was applied liberally
over the ear lobe for ~10 min. When applied, the cream rapidly heats up the
specific area and elicits a marked increase in blood flow. All arterialized blood
samples were measured in duplicate by the same investigator. The samples were
analyzed immediately (ABL 725, Radiometry, Copenhagen, London Scientific)
according to the manufacturer's instructions; the inter-assay coefficient of
variance was < 6%.

4.2.5   Statistical Analysis

Variables are presented as means ± standard deviation (SD). Data were initially
tested for normality, before being analysed by a one way repeated-measures
analysis of variance (ANOVA). The ANOVA results were corrected by the
Huynh-Feldt _-adjusted degrees of freedom when the violation to sphericity was
minimal (>0.75) and the Greenhouse-Geisser correction used when sphericity was
violated (<0.75), and significant condition and condition-time interactions were
identified (Field, 2001). Post hoc tests (Tukeys) were performed to isolate any

significant differences. Student's paired t-tests ascertained between-condition differences when a variable was measured once. For data which were not normally distributed, the Kruskal-Wallis test followed by the Wilcoxon matched-pair signed rank test, where appropriate, was used for analysis. Relationships between variables were examined using linear regression. Statistical significance was set at $P \leq 0.05$ for all statistical tests.

4.3   RESULTS

4.3.1   Subjects

All of the 12 subjects completed the 5 nights of normobaric hypoxia. One subject failed to complete the tests immediately following the hypoxic exposures and was withdrawn from the study; therefore, data from this subject was subsequently removed from the final analysis. The majority of the subjects reported initial discomfort, mild headaches and insomnia during the first night of hypoxic exposure; however, these symptoms became very mild during the subsequent 4 nights.

4.3.2   Resting Blood Samples and Related Variables

Mean values for the selected resting arterialized blood samples and related variables are given in Table 1. The coefficient-of-variance between control day 1 and control day 2 was < 6.5 %. Both PET_{CO_2} and arterialized P_{CO_2} (Pa_{CO_2}) showed a significant decrease (-3.5±1.9 Torr and –2.4±1.4 Torr, respectively; $P <$ 0.05) immediately following the hypoxic exposures, coinciding with increases in PET_{O_2} and arterialized P_{O_2} (Pa_{O_2}) (4.3±3.4 Torr and 2.7±5.2 Torr, respectively; P < 0.05) at this time point. When measured after 5 days of recovery, both the end-tidal gases and arterialized capillary samples had returned to control values. Although there was a marked trend for a progressive increase in hemoglobin and decrease in pH at following the exposure, this failed to reach significance ($P =$ 0.06 and $P = 0.072$, respectively). Likewise, base excess and bicarbonate tended to decrease, but due to large within group variance, failed to reach significance. The collective results from the arterialized capillary samples indicate that this method was quite successful in providing a useful estimate of arterial blood.

4.1
Mean values for the arterialized blood samples and related variables.

	Control 1	**Control 2**	**Day 3 of exposure**	**Day 1 Recovery**	**Day 5 Recovery**
Pa_{O_2}, Torr	78.2 ± 5.4	78.2 ± 4.0	78.4 ± 3.6	81.0 ± 3.4	75.6 ± 2.8*
Pa_{CO_2}, Torr	36.9 ± 2.0*	37.0 ± 2.0*	34.9 ± 2.0	34.5 ± 1.6	36.2 ± 2.6
[Hb], $g \cdot dl^{-1}$	16.1 ± 1.2	16.0 ± 1.2	17.1 ± 0.9	17.1 ± 1.3	16.5 ± 1.1
[HCO_3^-], $mmol \cdot l^{-1}$	24.0 ± 0.9	23.9 ± 1.2	23.3 ± 1.2	23.1 ± 1.2	23.3 ± 1.5
[$Base_{Ec}$], $mmol \cdot l^{-1}$	-0.83 ± 1.28	-0.63 ± 1.4	-1.87 ± 1.6	-2.1 ± 1.4	-1.75 ± 2.0
pH	7.411 ± 0.013	7.414 ± 0.007	7.416 ± 0.016	7.417 ± 0.012	7.406 ± 0.014
PET_{O_2}, Torr	86.5 ± 2.5**	86.0 ± 1.2**	NR	90.5 ± 2.6	87.6 ± 4.0
PET_{CO_2}, Torr	36.5 ± 1.1***	36.7 ± 1.2***	NR	33.1 ± 2.0	35.1 ± 1.8

Values are means ± SD. * denotes significant difference against day 1 recovery (* $P < 0.05$; ** $P < 0.01$; *** $P < 0.001$). Pa_{O_2} and Pa_{CO_2}, arterialized P_{O_2} and P_{CO_2}, respectively; Hb, hemoglobin concentration; HCO_3^-, standard bicarbonate concentration; $Base_{Ec}$, standard base excess concentration; PET_{O_2} and PET_{CO}, end-tidal P_{O_2} and P_{CO_2}; NR, not recorded.

4.3.3   Ventilatory Responses to Hypoxia and Hypercapnia

4.3.3.1   AHVR

A typical protocol for the determination of the AHVR, $\dot{V}_E$ hyperoxia and AHCVR is shown in Fig. 1. Mean values for these tests are given in Table 2. Immediately following the hypoxic exposure AHVR was increased by 1.6 ± 1.3 l·min^{-1}·%$^{-1}$ ($P < 0.01$) when compared with the control values (Fig. 2.). When tested at 5 days following the hypoxic exposure, the AHVR had returned back to control levels.

4.3.3.1 $\dot{V}_E$ hyperoxia and AHCVR:

There was a significant increase in ventilation when measured under conditions of hyperoxia ($P < 0.001$; Table 2). This increase in hyperoxic ventilation returned to control values when measured following the 5 days of recovery. Mean values for both the slope and intercept of the AHCVR are given in Table 2. These data are further illustrated in Fig. 3. There was a significant increase in the slope (1.5 ± 1.4 l·min^{-1}·Torr^{-1}; $P < 0.05$) and a decrease in the intercept (-2.7 ± 4.3 Torr; $P < 0.05$) of the AHCVR relationship. These changes in the AHCVR returned to baseline following 5 days of recovery. Collectively, the data indicate that 5 days recovery from the hypoxic exposure provided a suitable time frame during which AHVR, $\dot{V}_E$ hyperoxia and AHCVR returned to pre exposure values. In other words, the time course for both ventilatory acclimatization and de-acclimatization were very similar.

Figure 4.1

Sample breath-by-breath records for PET_{CO_2}, PET_{CO_2}, SaO_2 and ventilation

measured during an experimental determination of AHVR, $\dot{V}E$ hyperoxia and

AHCVR in subject 053 immediately following the 5 nights of normobaric

hypoxic exposure.

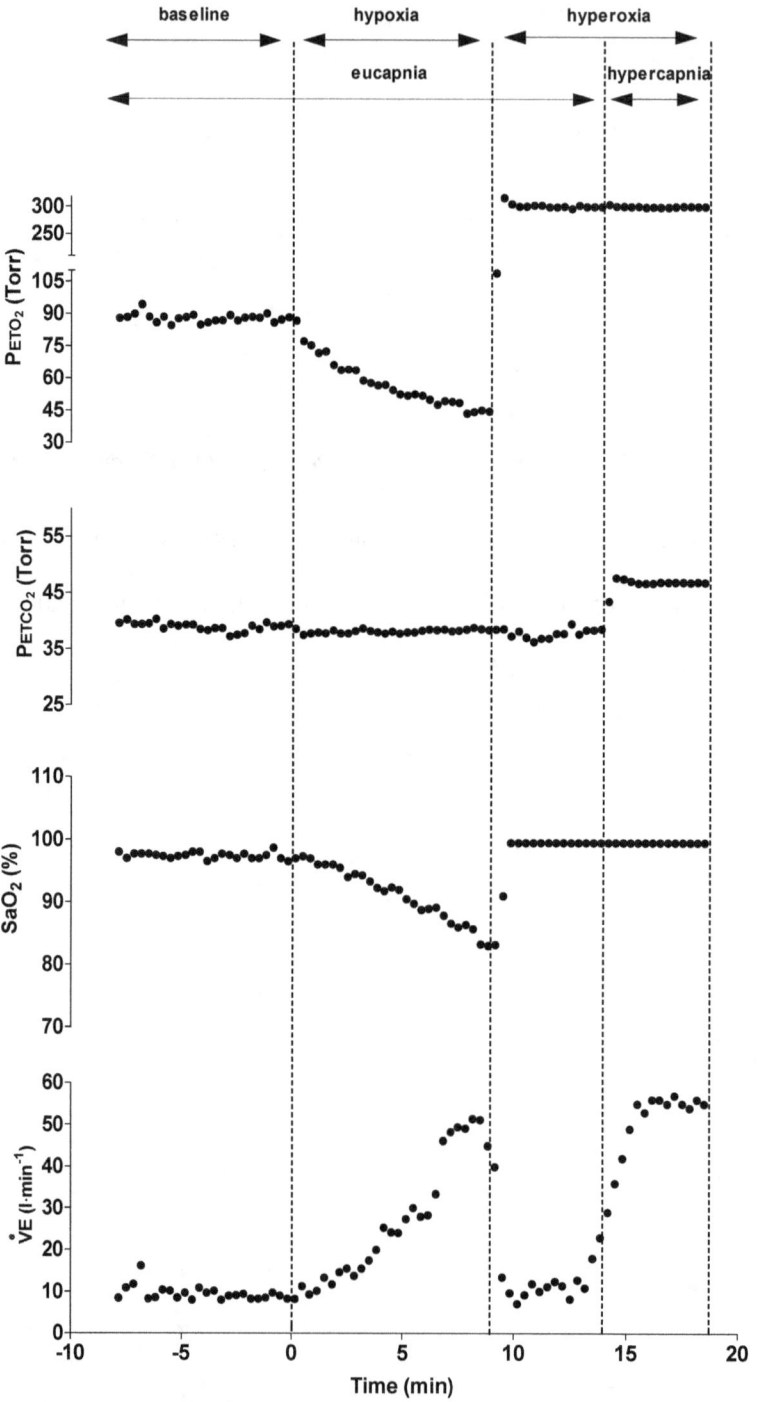

Figure 4.2

Acute hypoxic ventilatory response to isocapnic hypoxia (AHVR) prior to, and

following the 5 nights of normobaric hypoxia.

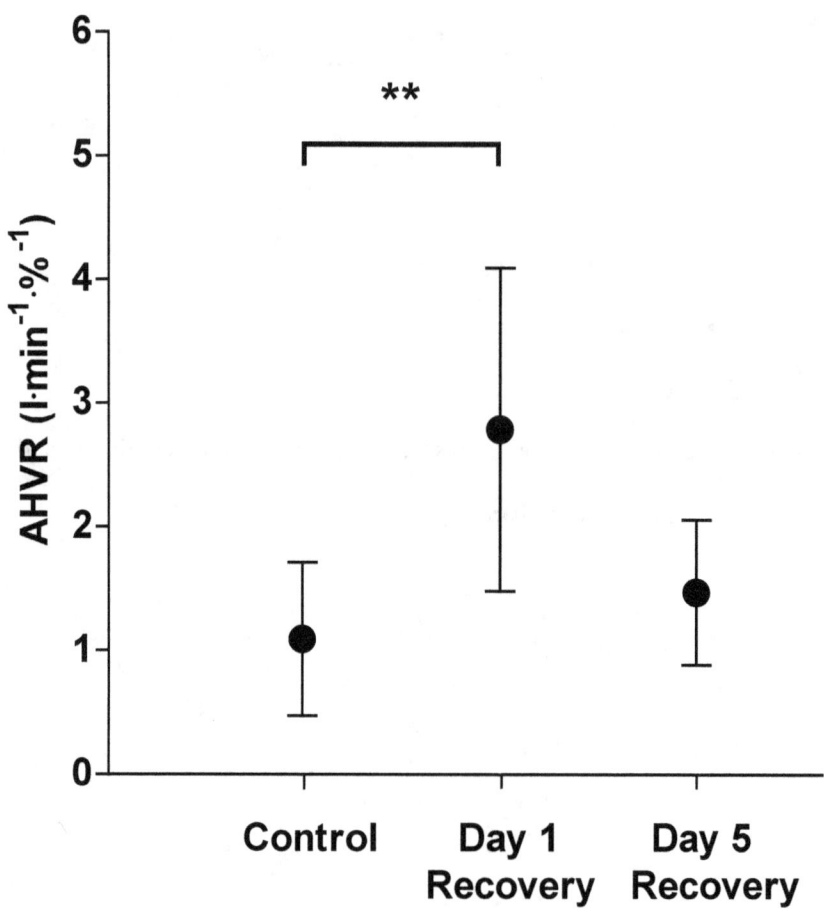

There were no marked differences in either the AHVR or AHCVR, in the 2 subjects who were measured at both their normal pre-exposure isocapnic clamp and during pH-matched conditions (data not shown). Interestingly, the slope of the AHCVR relationship was actually increased by 9% and 12% in the two subjects who were measured. Whilst only two subjects limit our speculation, this increase in the slope of the AHCVR is close to our reported day-to-day reproducibility of this measurement. Importantly, the data from these pH-matched tests suggest that they were no marked differences to that obtained from the $P_{ET_{CO_2}}$–clamped tests.

4.3.4 Relationships Between Selected Respiratory and Blood Variables

The significant decrease in the AHCVR intercept immediately following the hypoxic exposure was significantly correlated to: 1) the decrease in $P_{ET_{CO_2}}$ ($r = 0.55$; $P < 0.05$); 2) the increase in $P_{ET_{O_2}}$ ($r = -0.74$; $P < 0.05$); 3) the decrease in the estimated pH ($r = -0.681$; $P < 0.05$). Likewise, the increase in the slope of the AHCVR was correlated with the decrease in $P_{ET_{CO_2}}$ ($r = 0.40$; $P < 0.05$). The increase in the AHVR slope was significantly correlated to the increase in Pa_{O_2} ($r = 0.64$; $P < 0.05$). Furthermore, the decrease in $P_{ET_{CO_2}}$ following the exposure was correlated to the decrease in both pH ($r = -0.77$; $P < 0.05$) and HCO_3^- ($r = -0.772$; $P < 0.01$)

Figure 4.3

Ventilatory response to increases in $P_{ET_{CO_2}}$ during hyperoxic conditions prior to, and following the five nights of normobaric hypoxia.

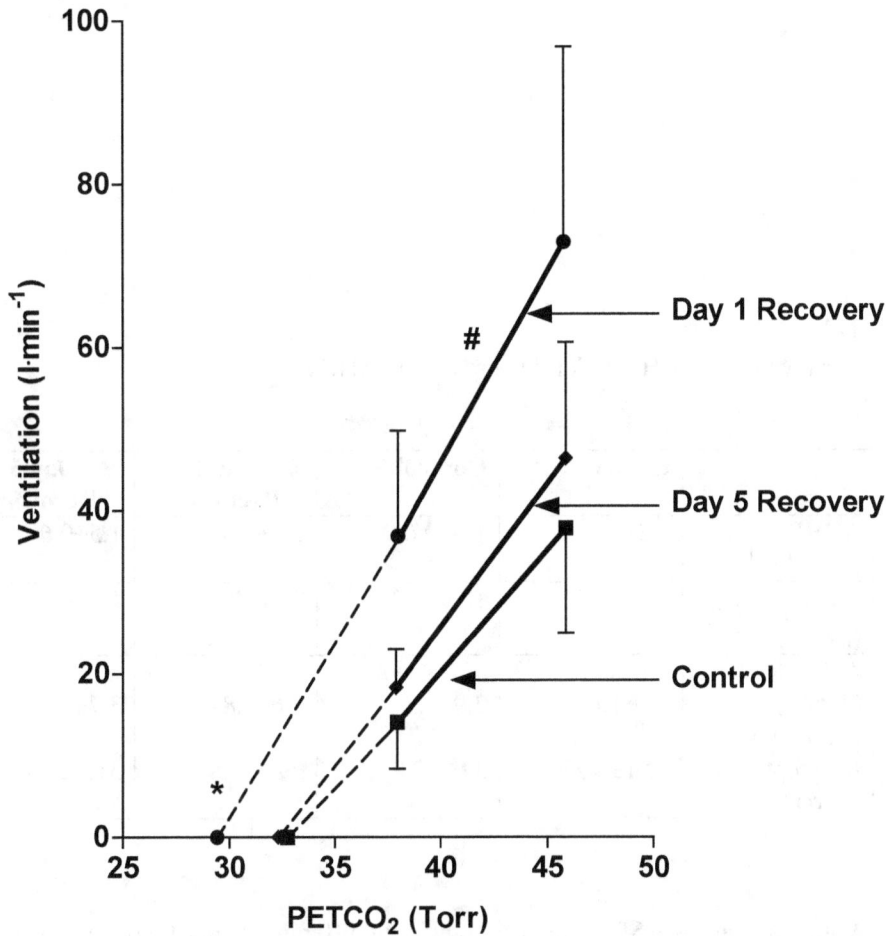

Table 4.2

Mean values for AHVR, $\dot{V}$E hyperoxia and AHCVR .

	Control 1	Control 5	Day 1 Recovery	Day 5 Recovery
AHVR ($l \cdot min^{-1} \cdot \%^{-1}$)	1.2±0.7**	1.0±0.6**	2.8±1.3	1.5±0.6
$\dot{V}$E hyperoxia ($l \cdot min^{-1}$)	10.3±3.6*	10.9±4.2	28.1±9.1	15.0±5.8
AHCVR Slope ($l \cdot min^{-1} \cdot Torr^{-1}$)	3.1±1.6*	2.9±1.2*	4.6±1.8	3.7±1.8
Intercept (Torr)	32.1±4.2*	32.3±3.8*	29.4±2.8	31.5±4.3

Values are means ± SD. * denotes significant difference against day 1 recovery

($* \; P < 0.05; ** \; P < 0.01$).

4.4   DISCUSSION

The present study has yielded a number of important and novel findings. Firstly, 5 nights of normobaric hypoxia elicited a pronounced increase in AHVR and leftward intercept shift of the AHCVR, together with an increase in the slope of this relationship. Such changes in the AHCVR following intermittent hypoxic exposure have not been shown previously. Secondly, the significant decrease in the $P_{ET_{CO_2}}$ following the hypoxic exposure was correlated both to the leftward intercept shift and an increase in the slope of the AHCVR. Finally, the time course for both ventilatory acclimatization and de-acclimatization were very similar. The following discussion details the assumptions and evidence that underlie these conclusions.

4.4.1   Methodological Considerations

4.4.1.1   *Isocapnic Respiratory Control Tests*

We chose to maintain $P_{ET_{CO_2}}$, for each subject, at ~1.5 Torr above their pre-exposure level; thus, although the isocapnia was different for each subject, it did not differ between tests. Numerous previous studies, using the end-tidal forcing technique, have used a similar protocol to assess the AHVR and AHCVR, and the data are comparable (Howard and Robbins, 1995; Tansley et al., 1998; Fatemain and Robbins, 1998; Fatemain and Robbins, 2001); however, one concern of this method is that the subjects, following the hypoxic exposure, are tested in a acute state of respiratory acidosis due to their $P_{ET_{CO_2}}$ being maintained at their pre-exposure level (J.A. Dempsey, personal communication to P.N. Ainslie). As a result, hyperoxic ventilation will be increased, at least in part, from the additional drive from the isocapnic P_{ETCO_2} clamp (2-8 Torr above resting following the hypoxic exposure). In addition, because P_{O_2} and P_{CO_2} interact at the peripheral chemoreceptors, the magnitude of the change in ventilation with hypoxia is critically dependent on the isocapnic level in this test; the higher the isocapnic P_{CO_2} above the resting P_{CO_2} the greater the AHVR (Severinghaus, 2001). Therefore, the decrease in the P_{ETCO_2} after hypoxic exposure could potentially account for some of the observed increase in the AHVR. Nevertheless, the ventilatory measurement recorded under hyperoxic conditions in the present study are almost identical to those reported after 48 hours of mild hypoxia after either isocapnic or poikilocapnic hypoxic conditions (Tansley et al., 1998).

In relation to the AHVR and AHCVR tests, two important points must be considered in support of the data and testing procedures. Firstly, the aforementioned study by Tansley et al. (1998) showed that the increases in the AHVR and the slope of the AHCVR did not differ following 48 hours isocapnic or poikilocapnic hypoxic conditions. In the same study, the AHVR and AHCVR measurements were conducted at both the pre-exposure P_{ETCO_2} level and also at a P_{ETCO_2} level matched for changes in arterial pH. The results did not differ between trials suggesting that, for mild hypoxic exposures over 48 hours, the pre-exposure P_{ETCO_2} clamp provided an equal assessment of the AHVR and AHCVR when compared to $P_{ET_{CO_2}}$-pH matched assessments. The pH-matched data obtained in the present study on 2 subjects also suggest that they were no marked differences to that obtained from the isocapnic tests conducted immediately following the hypoxic exposure.

Secondly, in order to account for a change in pH during hypoxic exposures, Severinghaus et al. (1966a) proposed that the AHCVR slopes obtained from altitude exposures can be standardized to sea level by multiplying the slope by the following factor: $(P_{CO_2} + 9)/49$, where P_{CO_2} is the normal altitude air breathing arterial value, 9 is the normal sea-level cerebrospinal fluid-to-arterial P_{CO_2} gradient, and 49 is normal sea-level cerebrospinal fluid P_{CO_2}). In the present study, this factor would be 0.856 (assuming the $P_{ET_{CO_2}}$ value of 33.1 Torr to be equal to Pa_{CO_2}). Corrected by this method, the slope of the AHCVR would still be 47%, as opposed to 55%, above that recorded during the control tests. In addition, when the between-test coefficient-of-variation (approximately 8%) is considered for the AHCVR, this increase in sensitivity of the slope, even when standardized to sea-level values, still represents a significant increase ($P < 0.05$). Ideally, following acclimatization to hypoxia, respiratory control tests should be carried out at a pH-matched level at the site of the central chemoreceptors as this is the pH level that matters for the AHCVR and it may differ from the arterial pH; however, data to resolve this issue is not obtainable. Finally, it should also be pointed out that the respiratory control tests, as used in the present study, do not discriminate between a change in the interaction of P_{CO_2} and P_{O_2} at the peripheral chemoreceptors and an increase in overall peripheral chemoreceptor activity.

4.4.1.2 Timing of the Respiratory Control Tests

Immediately following the AHVR, subjects were exposed to 5 minutes of hyperoxia ($P_{ET_{O_2}} = 300$ Torr) in an attempt to minimize any prior effects of the hypoxia. Whether or not this brief hypoxic exposure may influence the AHCVR test is unclear. Nevertheless, all test were conducted using the exact same protocol, and the AHCVR data are consist with previous values obtained from chronic altitude studies (Michel and Milledge, 1963; Forster et al., 1971). Finally, since there is a known circadian rhythm on respiratory control (Stephenson et al., 2000), all tests were conducted at the same time of day, within 2 hours of the subjects leaving the hypoxic exposures.

4.4.1.3 Experimental Design:

The experimental design incorporated in the present study was a one-group time series design i.e., subjects visited the laboratory 3 times prior to the hypoxic intervention in order to establish the reproducibility of the control measurements. If the reproducibility of the measured variables is high, this type of experimental design provides as valid alterative to inclusion of a control group (Campbell and Stanley, 1966). We are confident in the use of such a design, and of our results, as the reproducibility of our control measurements are very high and the increases in the ventilatory responses are significant when the subsequent coefficients of variations are considered into the analysis.

4.4.2   Ventilatory Responses to Hypoxia and Hypercapnia

4.4.2.1   Change in AHCVR:
To the best of our knowledge, this study is the first to show a leftward intercept shift of the ventilatory response to an increase in $P_{ET_{CO_2}}$, together with an increase in the slope of this relationship, following an intermittent hypoxic exposure. The major reasons why previous intermittent hypoxic studies (Katayama et al., 1998) and a number of chamber studies (Howard and Robbins, 1995; Tansley et al., 1998; Fatemian and Robbins, 1998; Fatemian and Robbins, 2001) have failed to note any change in the AHCVR are most likely due to the level of hypoxia being too moderate and/or the duration of exposure being to short. For example, Schoene et al. (1990) have demonstrated that AHCVR did not increase at barometric pressure of 452 Torr, while it did increase at 305 Torr. Furthermore, no human or animal studies have shown changes in the AHCVR intercept following periods of isocapnic hypoxia. It would therefore seem probable that respiratory alkalosis is required to generate significant changes in the AHCVR relationship. The requirement of respiratory alkalosis to generate changes in the AHCVR intercept is supported by studies at high altitude (Hasselbalch and Lindhard, 1911; Kellogg et al., 1957; Forster et al., 1971; White et al., 1987) and from a recent hyperventilation study (Ren and Robbins, 1999). In the latter study, utilizing the dynamic end-tidal forcing technique, the leftward

intercept shift in the AHCVR relationship following 6 h of passive hyperventilation was due to alkalosis and not hyperventilation when alkalosis was subsequently prevented (Ren and Robbins, 1999). The lack of AHCVR intercept shifts with isocapnia (Howard and Robbins, 1995; Tansley et al., 1998), and the finding of such a shift with poikilocapnia (Hasselbalch and Lindhard, 1911; Kellogg et al., 1957; Forster et al., 1971; White et al., 1987), argue in favor of the acid-base changes accounting for the shift. However, the data from the aforementioned hyperventilation study also showed that the increase in the slope of the AHCVR relationship was due to the hyperventilation per se and not the hypocapnia (Ren and Robbins, 1999). Whilst these data are interesting, due to the relatively short time frame of the hyperventilation (6 hours), we accept the possibility that central acid base changes may explain both the shift in the intercept and also an increase in the slope of the AHCVR.

Our findings differ from those observed by the Toronto group (Mahamed and Duffin, 2001; Mahamed et al., 2003), who observed no change in the sensitivity of the AHCVR, following either repeated 20 min daily exposures to hypoxia over 14 days (Mahamed and Duffin, 2001) or to 3 hours of isocapnic hypoxia (Mahamed et al., 2003). After both exposures, a decrease in the threshold for the ventilatory response to carbon dioxide during hypoxic rebreathing tests was observed. This difference in findings could be due to both methodological differences and also due to the shorter length of the exposure; 3 h compared with

8-9 h·day^{-1} overnight for 5 days. One possibility is that a change in the threshold of the ventilatory response to carbon dioxide requires only very brief periods of hypoxia (Mahamed and Duffin, 2001; Mahamed et al., 2003), whereas an increase in the sensitivity is only apparent after a longer duration of (>7 h) mild hypoxia (Fatemian and Robbins, 1998; Tansley et al., 1998; Fatemian and Robbins, 2001). In support of this notion, Tansley et al. (1998) suggest that the increase in the slope of the AHCVR begins early in ventilatory acclimatization to hypoxia but that changes in intercept require a longer duration of hypoxia, a more intense level of hypoxia, or a shift in the acid-base status of the blood. The possibility that a change in the threshold of the AHCVR precedes, or is required for a change in the slope of the AHCVR, remains to be explored.

In the present study, the decrease in PET_{CO_2} after the hypoxic exposure was correlated to the leftward intercept shift and the slope of the AHCVR relationship. Although not cause and effect, one possible explanation for these relationships may be associated with the changes in PET_{CO_2}, and hence Pa_{CO_2}, reflecting an acid-base affect that is likely to be related to the stimulus at the central chemoreceptors. For example, the resulting hypocapnia would likely lead to decreases in the bicarbonate concentration in the interstitial space of the brain and the cerebrospinal fluid (Fencl, 1986). Likewise, there is evidence to suggest that hypocapnia can also cause bicarbonate depletion, via an increase in lactate production within the brain (Fencl, 1986). Since the stimulus at the central chemoreceptors is influenced, in part, by the cerebrospinal fluid (Pappenheimer et al., 1965), the lowered bicarbonate concentration and, providing the P_{CO_2} is the same, the lower pH, after the hypoxic exposure, will provide a greater respiratory stimulus (Dempsey et al., 1975). These possible changes around the central chemoreceptors, mediated by the hypocapnia, may be one potential mechanism to explain the shift in the AHCVR.

A second possible explanation for the AHCVR results is based the feature of the steady-state technique to underestimate the response slope because the end-tidal to brain tissue (extracelluar) P_{CO_2} difference decreases as P_{CO_2} increases (Pandit et al., 2003). Some studies (Severinghaus et al., 1966b), but not all (Moller et al., 2002; Poulin et al., 2002), have shown cerebral blood flow to increase following hypoxic exposures. If we assume that cerebral blood flow has increased (Severinghaus et al., 1966b) and sensitivity to P_{O_2} and P_{CO_2} has also increased (Poulin et al., 2002) following the hypoxic exposure, then the relation between the end-tidal to brain tissue P_{CO_2} difference and P_{CO_2} during AHCVR test will be altered and may produce a decrease in the underestimation of the response slope, i.e. an increase in AHCVR slope and a decrease in intercept.

4.4.2.2   Change in AHVR
Our results further support the large body of literature that hypoxic exposures induces large increases in AHVR, as previously reported during natural

acclimatization (Forster et al., 1971; Reeves et al., 1993; Sato et al., 1994), after a range of intermittent exposures (Levine et al. 1992; Katayama et al., 1998; Garcia et al., 2000; Townsend et al., 2002), and 8 h of very mild hypoxia (Fatemian et al., 2001). Our findings for AHVR from this cohort of subjects are representative with those reported by others (Levine et al., 1992; Howard and Robbins, 1995; Katayama et al., 1998; Garcia et al., 2000; Tansley et al., 1998; Townsend et al., 2002). Recent investigations in humans (Howard and Robbins, 1995; Tansley et al., 1998), utilizing isocapnic hypoxic conditions, suggest that increases in AHVR seem to depend on the hypoxia *per se* and not on the presence of respiratory alkalosis.

Reeves et al. (1993) provide data to show that PET_{CO_2} values and the AHVR as measured at sea level is related to the extent of subsequent ventilatory acclimatization (decrease in PET_{CO_2}) and the level of oxygenation at altitude on arrival and after 19 days residence at 4,300 m. More recently, Townsend et al. (2002) showed similar relationships between sea level AHVR and the decrease in PET_{CO_2} after 1 and 3 nights of intermittent hypoxic exposure (~2,650m). In contrast to the aforementioned investigations by Reeves et al. (1993) and Townsend et al. (2002), we did not find any correlations between the control AHVR and changes in PET_{CO_2}. The disparity in these results might be related to the different techniques used to measure AHVR, and to the different duration and intensity of the hypoxic exposures.

It is unfortunate that the investigations by Reeves et al. (1993) and Townsend et al. (2002) did not measure the AHCVR. As mentioned, the leftward shift in the AHCVR relationship has been suggested to be related to the degree of re-setting of the central chemoreceptors to start responding to a lowered P_{CO_2}. Therefore, the relationship between the decrease in $P_{ET_{CO_2}}$ and the leftward shift of the AHCVR may provide more of a meaningful indication of ventilatory acclimatization [i.e. a change in the P_{CO_2} set point of the respiratory control mechanism; (Cunnningham et al., 1986)] than the AHVR alone.

In summary, this study described the effects of 5 nights of normobaric hypoxia on the acute ventilatory responses to isocapnic hypoxia and to hyperoxic hypercapnia. The data support the notion that intermittent hypoxia, at a simulated attitude of 4300 m, can elicit similar perturbations in the ventilatory responses to both hypoxia and hypercapnia to that shown during more chronic altitude exposure.

4.5   REFERENCES

Campbell, D.T., Stanley, J. C., 1966. Experimental and Quasi-experimental Designs for Research, Rand McNally and Company, Chicago.

Cunnningham, D.J.C., Robbins, P.A., Wolf, C.B., 1986. Integration of respiratory responses to changes in alveolar partial pressures of CO_2 and O_2 and in arterial pH. In: Fishman, A.P. Handbook of Physiology, Section 3: The Respiratory System, Vol. II, Part 2: Control of Breathing. American Physiology Society, Bethesda, MD, pp. 475-528.

Dempsey, J.A., Forster, H.V., Gledhill, N., DoPico, G.A., 1975. Effects of moderate hypoxemia and hypocapnia on CSF [H^+] and ventilation in man. Journal of Applied Physiology 38, 665-674.

Dempsey, J.A., Forster, H.V., 1982. Mediation of ventilatory adaptations. Physiological Reviews 62, 262-346.

Fatemian, M., Robbins, P.A., 1998. Human ventilatory response to CO_2 after 8 h of isocapnic or poikilocapnic hypoxia. Journal of Applied Physiology 85, 1922-1928.

Fatemian, M., Kim, D.Y., Poulin, M.J., Robbins, P.A., 2001. Very mild exposure to hypoxia for 8 h can induce ventilatory acclimatization in humans. Pflügers Archiv 441, 840-843.

Fatemian, M., Robbins, P.A., 2001. Selected contribution: chemoreflex responses to CO_2 before and after an 8 h exposure to hypoxia in humans. Journal of Applied Physiology 90, 1607-1614.

Field, A., 2000. Discovering Statistics using SPSS for Windows. Cromwell Press, London.

Fencl, V., 1986. Acid-base balance in cerebral fluids. In: Fishman, A.P. Handbook of Physiology, Section 3: The Respiratory System, Vol. II, Part 1: Control of Breathing. American Physiology Society, Bethesda, MD, pp. 115-140.

Forster, H.V., Dempsey, J.A., Birnbaum, M.L., Reddan, W.G., Thoden, J., Grover, R.F., Rankin, J., 1971. Effect of chronic exposure to hypoxia on ventilatory response to CO_2 and hypoxia. Journal of Applied Physiology 31, 586-592.

Garcia, N., Hopkins, S.R., Powell, F.L., 2000. Effects of intermittent hypoxia on the isocapnic ventilatory response and erythropoiesis in humans. Respiration Physiology 123, 39-49.

Hasselbalch, K.A., Lindhard, J., 1911. Analyse des höhenklimas in seinen wirkungen auf die respiration. Skandinavisches Archiv für Physiologie 25, 361-408.

Howard, L.S.G.E., Robbins, P.A., 1995. Alterations in respiratory control during eight hours of isocapnic and poikilocapnic hypoxia in humans. Journal of Applied Physiology 78, 1098-1107.

Howson, M.G., Khamnei, S., McIntyre, M. E., O'Connor, D.F., Robbins, P.A., 1987. A rapid computer controlled binary gas mixing system for studies in respiratory control. Journal of Physiology, London, 394, 7P.

Ide, K., Eliasziw, M., Poulin, M. J., 2003. The relationship between middle cerebral artery blood velocity and end-tidal P_{CO_2} in the hypocapnic-hypercapnic range in humans. Journal of Applied Physiology 95: 129-137.

Katayama, K., Sato, Y., Ishida, K., Mori, S., Miyamura, M., 1998. The effects of intermittent exposure to hypoxia during endurance training on the ventilatory responses to hypoxia and hypercapnia in humans. European Journal of Applied Physiology 78, 189-194.

Kellogg, R.H., Pace, N., Archibald, E.R., Vaughan, B.E., 1957. Respiratory responses to inspired CO_2 during acclimatization to an altitude of 12,470 feet. Journal of Applied Physiology 11, 65-71.

Levine, B.D., Friedman, D.B., Engfred, K., Hanel, B., Kjaer, M., Clifford, P.S., Secher, N.H., 1992. The effect of normoxic or hypobaric hypoxic training on the hypoxic ventilatory response. Medicine and Science in Sports and Exercise 24, 769-775.

Michel, C.C., Milledge, J.S., 1963. Respiratory regulation in man during acclimatization to high altitude. Journal of Physiology, London, 168, 631-643.

Mahamed, S., Duffin, J., 2001. Repeated hypoxic exposures change respiratory chemoreflex control in humans. Journal of Physiology, London, 534, 595-603.

Mahamed, S., Cunningham, D.A, Duffin, J., 2003. Changes in respiratory control after three hours of isocapnic hypoxia in humans. Journal of Physiology, London, 547, 271-281.

Michel, C.C., Lloyd, B.B., Cunningham, D.J.C., 1966. The in vivo carbon dioxide dissociation curve of true plasma. Respirpiration Physiology 1, 121-137.

Moller, K., Paulson, O.B., Hornbein, T.F., Colier, W.N., Paulson, A.S., Roach, R.C., Holm, S., Knudsen, G.M., 2002. Unchanged cerebral blood flow and oxidative metabolism after acclimatization to high altitude. Journal of Cerebral Blood Flow and Metabolism 22, 118-26.

Mou, X. B., Howard, L. S., Robbins, P. A., 1995. A protocol for determining the shape of the ventilatory response to hypoxia in humans. Respiration Physiology 101, 139-143.

Pandit, J.J., Mohan, R.M., Paterson, N.D., Poulin., M.J., 2003. Cerebral blood flow sensitivity to CO_2 measured with steady-state and Read's rebreathing methods. Respiration Physiology and Neurobiology *In press.*

Pappenheimer, J.R., Fencl, V., Heisey, S.R., Held, D., 1965. Role of cerebral fluids in control of respiration as studied in anaesthetized goats. American Journal of Physiology 208, 436-450.

Poulin, M.J., Fatemian, M., Tansley, J.G., O'Connor, D.F., Robbins, P.A., 2002. Changes in cerebral blood flow during and after 48 h of both isocapnic and poikilocapnic hypoxia in humans. Experimental Physiology 87, 633-42.

Reeves, J.T., McCullough, R.E., Moore, L.G., Cymerman, A., Weil, J.V., 1993. Sea-level PCO_2 relates to ventilatory acclimatization at 4,300m. Journal of Applied Physiology 75, 1117-1122.

Ren, X., Robbins, P.A., 1999. Ventilatory responses to hypercapnia and hypoxia after 6 h passive hyperventilation in humans. Journal of Physiology, London, 514, 885-894.

Robbins, P.A., Swanson, G.D., Howson, M.G., 1982. A prediction correction scheme for forcing alveolar gases along certain time courses. Journal of Applied Physiology 52, 1353-1357.

Sato, M., Severinghaus, J.W., Bickler, P., 1994. Time course of augmentation and depression of hypoxic ventilatory response at altitude. Journal of Applied Physiology 77, 313-316.

Schoene, R.B., Roach, R.C., Hackett, P.H., Sutton, J.R., Cymerman, A., Houston, C.S., 1990. Operation Everest II: ventilatory adaptation during gradual decompression to extreme altitude. Medicine and Science in Sports and Exercise 22, 804-810.

Severinghaus, J.W., Bainton, C.R., Carcelen, A., 1966a. Respiration insensitivity to hypoxia in chronically hypoxic man. Respiration Physiology 1, 308-334.

Severinghaus, J.W., Chiodi, H., Eger, E.I., Brandstater, B., Hornbein, T.F., 1966b. Cerebral blood flow in man at high altitude. Role of cerebrospinal fluid pH in normalization of flow in chronic hypocapnia. Circulation Research 19, 274-282.

Severinghaus, J.W., 1977. Simple, accurate equations for human blood O_2 dissociation computations. Journal of Applied Physiology 46, 599-602.

Severinghaus, J. W., 2001. Cerebral circulation at high altitude. In: Hornbein, T.F., Schoene, R. B. High Altitude: An Exploration of Human Adaptation. Marcel Dekker, New York, pp. 343-375.

Stephenson, R., Mohan, R.M., Duffin, J., Jarsky, T.M., 2000. Circadian rhythms in the chemoreflex control of breathing. American Journal of Physiology 278, R282-286.

Tansley, J.G., Fatemian, M., Howard, L.S.G.E., Poulin, M.J., Robbins, P.A., 1998. Changes in respiratory control during and after 48 h of isocapnic and poikilocapnic hypoxia in humans. Journal of Applied Physiology 85, 2125-2134.

Townsend, N.E., Gore, C.J., Hahn, A.G., McKenna, M.J., Aughey, R.J., Clark, S.A., Kinsman, T., Hawley, J.A., Chow, C-M., 2002. Living high-training low increases hypoxic ventilatory response of well-trained endurance athletes. Journal of Applied Physiology 93, 1498-1505.

White, D.P., Glesson, K., Pickett, C.K., Rannels, A.M., Cymerman, A., Weil, J.V., 1987. Altitude acclimatization: influence on periodic breathing and chemoresponsiveness during sleep. Journal of Applied Physiology 63, 401-412.

CHAPTER 5

EFFECTS OF 5 CONSECUTIVE NOCTURNAL

HYPOXIC EXPOSURES ON THE

CEREBROVASCULAR RESPONSES TO ACUTE

HYPOXIA AND HYPERCAPNIA IN HUMANS

5.1   INTRODUCTION

In humans, cerebral blood flow (CBF) increases in response to acute hypoxia (Kety and Schmidt, 1948; Severinghaus et al., 1966; Huang et al., 1987; Poulin et al., 2002). The magnitude of the CBF response to hypoxia is dependent on the balance between the hypoxemic induced cerebrovasodilatation and the cerebral vasoconstriction secondary to hypocapnia associated with the increased ventilation (Schoene, 1999; Severinghaus, 2001). Over the course of several days, the process of ventilatory acclimatization to the hypoxia of altitude unfolds and the degree of hypoxemia is reduced, while the degree of hypocapnia increases (Severinghaus et al., 1966; Jensen et al., 1996). Several studies (Buck et al., 1998; Jansen et al., 1999; Roach and Hackett, 2001) have reported that the interaction between these opposing vascular reflexes may contribute to individual susceptibility to altitude diseases such as acute mountain sickness (AMS) and high altitude cerebral edema (HACE).

To address the issue of whether the cerebrovascular sensitivity to hypoxia was altered during the process of acclimatization, Jensen et al. (Jensen et al., 1996) quantified the CBF responses in humans during a high altitude field study. Over a 5 day sojourn at altitude (3810m), Jensen and colleagues reported that the sensitivity of CBF to acute variations in isocapnic hypoxia increased 34%, while the CBF sensitivity to acute variations in hypercapnia increased 28%. Similar increases in CBF sensitivities to acute variations in O_2 and CO_2 have recently been reported by Poulin et al. (Poulin et al., 2002) following 48 hours of continuous isocapnic and poikilocapnic hypoxic exposures in humans. While these studies and others (Severinghaus et al., 1966; Otis et al., 1989; Jensen et al., 1996; Jansen et al., 1999) have examined the effect of chronic hypoxia on cerebral vasomotor reactivity, the impact of discontinuous hypoxia on cerebrovascular events has received little attention. The aim of the present study was to establish a discontinuous hypoxic intervention that would elicit physiological perturbations comparable to those observed during adaptation to chronic hypoxia. We hypothesized that 5 consecutive overnight normobaric hypoxic exposures (8 hours / night) at a simulated altitude of 4300m would elicit similar changes in cerebrovascular sensitivities to acute hypoxia and hypercapnia to those reported during chronic altitude exposures. Additionally, there have been reports that alterations in regional cerebral oxygen saturation (S_rO_2) may be associated with the cerebrovascular response to chronic hypoxia (Imray et al., 1998; Saito et al., 1999). Therefore we simultaneously measured S_rO_2 to gain further insight regarding the role cerebral oxygenation may have on CBF sensitivities before and after the 5 consecutive nocturnal hypoxic exposures. This cerebrovascular study was undertaken in conjunction with a study examining the ventilatory responses to nocturnal hypoxia (Ainslie et al., 2003).

5.2 METHODS

5.2.1 Subjects

Twelve healthy male subjects (26.6 ± 4.1 (SD) yrs) participated in this study. The requirements of the study were fully explained to all subjects, with each subject giving written informed consent before participating in the study. The research project was approved by the University of Calgary Conjoint Health Research Ethics Board. All subjects were non-smokers, none was taking any medication, and none of the subjects had any history of respiratory, cardiovascular or cerebrovascular disease. Prior to commencing the main experimental procedures, each subject made a preliminary visit to the laboratory which served as a familiarization session to the laboratory and apparatus. During this initial visit, measurements of resting end-tidal gases and estimates of hypoxic and hypercapnic sensitivities were conducted. The laboratory is located at an altitude of 1103 m above sea level and the average barometric pressure for the duration of the study was 667 ± 14 Torr.

5.2.2 Protocol

The experimental design, illustrating the timing of measurements, and the sequence of nocturnal hypoxic exposures, is presented in Table 1. One week prior to the nocturnal hypoxic exposures, each subject participated in a control sleep under normoxic conditions to obtain overnight baseline measurements.

Timing and sequence of experimental measurements	CS	C1	C5	E1	E2	E3	E4	E5	R1	R5
				Nocturnal Hypoxic Exposures						
Overnight measurements										
• SaO_2	√			√	√	√	√	√		
• PET_{CO_2}	√			√	√	√	√	√		
• AMS symptoms	√			√	√	√	√	√		
Blood measurements										
• Evening (normoxia)	√			√	√	√	√	√		
• Morning (normoxia)	√									√
• Morning (hypoxia)				√	√	√	√	√		
Dynamic Measurements										
• Sensitivity of CBF to acute variations in hypoxia		√	√						√	√
• Sensitivity of CBF to acute variations in CO_2		√	√						√	√
• Sensitivity of SrO_2 to acute variations in hypoxia		√	√						√	√
• Sensitivity of SrO_2 to acute variations in CO_2		√	√						√	√

Table 5.1

Overnight measurements made inside the hypoxic chamber during the nocturnal hypoxic exposures: SaO_2, arterial oxygen saturation (pulse oximetry); PET_{CO_2}, end-tidal PCO_2; AMS symptoms, Lake Louise Acute Mountain Sickness Scoring System. Blood measurements for E1 - E5 were made before entering the chamber (normoxia) and in the morning following 8 hr of hypoxia prior to exiting the chamber. Dynamic cerebrovascular measurements were made before and after the 5 consecutive overnight hypoxic exposures using an end-tidal forcing system to control the end-tidal gases. Abbreviations: CS, control sleep (normoxia); C1 and C5, control day 1 and control day 5; E1 - E5, overnight exposures to hypoxia; R1 and R5, recovery day 1 and recovery day 5 following E1 - E5.

Subsequently, each subject reported to the laboratory on two occasions, 5 days apart, at the same time of day following an overnight fast for control measurements of the sensitivity of CBF and S_rO_2 to an acute incremental hypoxic protocol using an end-tidal forcing system to control end-tidal gases. Following the final control measurement, each subject underwent 5 consecutive over-night sleep exposures of normobaric hypoxia at a simulated altitude of ~ 4300m (F_IO_2 ~ 13.8%; P_IO_2 ~ 88 Torr). Immediatley following the 5 nocturnal hypoxic exposures, and after 5 days of recovery, subjects reported to the laboratory to repeat the measurements of cerebrovascular sensitivities to acute variations in hypoxia and CO_2.

5.2.3   Nocturnal Hypoxic Exposures and Overnight Measurements

Subjects entered the purpose-designed chambers (Hypoxico, Inc) at approximately 2300 hrs and exited at 0700 hrs the following morning. Between the nocturnal hypoxic exposures (~ 16 h normoxia), subjects maintained their normal daily activities. Throughout the control sleep and all overnight hypoxic exposures, pulse oximetry (Nellcor N-295, Nellcor Inc., Hayward, CA, USA) was used to continuously monitor arterial oxygen saturation (SaO_2) (Kolb et al., 2003). Prior to entering the chamber, subjects were fitted with a fine nasal catheter which was connected to a CO_2 analyzer (Normocap-Oxy Monitor, Datex-Ohmeda, Mississauga, Ontario, Canada) for determining overnight end-tidal PCO_2 values.

End-tidal PCO_2 values were measured and averaged over a 5 minute period each hour throughout each night.

Blood measurements were conducted each night prior to entering the chamber and following 8 h of hypoxia prior to exiting the chamber. Micro blood samples (~200µl) were obtained by finger tip penetration and immediately analyzed for blood gases (PO_2 and PCO_2), hemoglobin, and hematocrit using an i-STAT Portable Clinical Analyzer (G6+ cartridge, i-STAT Corp., Princeton, NJ, USA). After the 5 intermittent hypoxic exposures subjects were permitted to go home, but were asked to maintain their normal diet and physical activity levels.

The presence and severity of the AMS symptoms of headache, gastrointestinal upset, fatigue or weakness, dizziness, and difficulty sleeping were evaluated with the Lake Louise Acute Mountain Sickness Scoring System questionnaire (Roach et al., 1993). Each symptom was evaluated on a sliding scale ranging from 0 (no symptom) to 3 (severe). The diagnostic criteria for AMS, as outlined in the scoring system, stipulates the presence of headache and any other symptom(s). A summated score of three or more constitutes the incidence of moderate AMS. The questionnaire was completed by each subject at the beginning of each overnight session, after four hours, and after eight hours prior to exiting the chamber.

5.2.4   Incremental Step Hypoxic and Hypercapnic Protocol

Subjects reported to the laboratory at the same time each morning following an overnight fast. On each of these visits, the subject's normal end-tidal PO_2 (PET_{O_2}) and end-tidal PCO_2 (PET_{CO_2}) values were measured prior to the experiment, while the subject was sitting quietly and comfortably for approximately 10 min. The respired gases were sampled via a fine catheter held at the opening of one nostril by an adapted nasal O_2 therapy kit. The gas was sampled continuously at a rate of 20 ml·min^{-1} and analyzed for PO_2 and PCO_2 by mass spectrometer (AMIS 2000, Innovision, Odense, Denmark). Values for PO_2 and PCO_2 were sampled by computer every 10ms. PET_{O_2} and PET_{CO_2} were identified and recorded for each breath using a computer and dedicated software (Chamber v1.00, University Laboratory of Physiology, Oxford, UK).

The experimental protocol began with an eight-minute period during which the subject breathed normally through a mouthpiece with the nose occluded by a nose clip. Respiratory volumes and flow information were obtained with a pneumotachograph and differential pressure transducer (RSS100-HR, Hans Rudolf Inc., Kansas City, MO, USA). Respiratory flow direction and timing information were measured with a turbine volume transducer (VMM-400, Interface Associates, CA, USA). Accurate control of the end-tidal gases was achieved using the technique of dynamic end-tidal forcing (BreatheM v2.07, University Laboratory of Physiology, Oxford, UK). A controlling computer generated the inspired partial pressure of O_2 and CO_2 predicted to give the desired end-tidal partial pressures by using a fast gas mixing system (Robbins et al., 1982; Howson et al., 1987). The controlling computer received feedback of the measured end-tidal partial pressures on a breath-by-breath basis as the experiment progressed. These measured end-tidal values were compared with the desired values, and the computer then adjusted the initial predicted inspired gas mixture by using an integral proportional feedback algorithm based on the deviations of the measured end-tidal values from the desired end-tidal values (Robbins et al., 1982).

The hypoxic stimulus was varied by holding the $P_{ET_{O_2}}$ at 7 different predetermined levels over the range of 88-45 Torr while the $P_{ET_{CO_2}}$ was held constant at eucapnia (1.5 Torr above the subject's initial air-breathing value before the start of the overnight hypoxic exposures). These levels were calculated to provide equal steps in oxygen saturation of the arterial blood, by using the relationship described by Severinghaus (Severinghaus, 1979). An eight-minute lead in period consisted of eucapnic euoxia ($P_{ET_{O_2}}$ = 88 Torr) followed by 6 descending steps ($P_{ET_{O_2}}$ = 75.2, 64.0, 57.0, 52.0, 48.2, and 45.0 Torr), each step lasting 90 sec. Immediately after the last step, $P_{ET_{O_2}}$ was elevated to 300 Torr for 5 min while $P_{ET_{CO_2}}$ remained at eucapnia. Then, $P_{ET_{CO_2}}$ was raised an additional 7.5 Torr for 5 min whilst $P_{ET_{O_2}}$ remained constant at 300 Torr. The final ten minutes of this protocol served to establish the changes in the cerebrovascular responses to hypercapnia.

5.2.5 Measurement of Cerebral Oxygenation

Throughout the experimental protocol, near-infrared spectroscopy was used to monitor cerebral oxygenation (S_rO_2) in the brain (INVOS 4100, TYCO Health Care Group Canada Inc., Pointe-Claire, QC, Canada). A light emitting diode (SomaSensor, Tyco Health Care Group Canada Inc.) was carefully placed over the right front-temporal region of the forehead, just above the eyebrow and left of the midsaggital sulcus. The SomaSensor alternately generates two wavelengths of light (730 and 805nm) which detect oxygenated and deoxygenated states of hemoglobin to estimate an index of oxygen saturation based on internal micro-processing algorithms (Kim et al., 2000). Analogue signals of S_rO_2 were obtained every 2 sec throughout the protocol and stored for later analysis.

5.2.6 Measurement of Cerebral Blood Flow

Backscattered Doppler signals from the right middle cerebral artery (MCA) were measured continuously during the protocol using a 2MHz pulsed Doppler Ultrasound system (TC22, SciMed, Bristol, England). The MCA was identified by an insonation pathway through the right temporal window just above the zygomatic arch by using search techniques described previously (Poulin and Robbins, 1996). The Doppler probe was secured with a headband device (Müller and Moll Fixation, Nicolet Instruments, Madison, Wisconsin, USA) to maintain optimal insonation position and angle throughout the protocol. In this study, the peak blood velocity (VP) was acquired every 10ms and averaged over each heart beat ($\overline{VP}$), and this was used as the primary index of CBF (Poulin and Robbins, 1996).

5.2.7   Sensitivity of CBF and S_rO_2 to Acute Variations of P_{ETO_2} and P_{ETCO_2}

The acute hypoxic CBF response (AHRCBF) was determined by linear regression between the mean $\overline{VP}$ and arterial oxygen saturation (100-SaO$_2$) during the final 20 s of each incremental step of hypoxia. Similarly, the acute hypoxic cerebral oxygenation response (AHRS$_rO_2$) was determined by linear regression between S_rO_2 and arterial oxygen saturation during the final 20 sec of each hypoxic step. The acute hypercapnic CBF response (AHCRCBF) and the acute hypercapnic cerebral oxygenation response (AHCRS$_rO_2$) were determined by linear regression between the mean $\overline{VP}$ and S$_rO_2$ respectively, during the final minute of the hyperoxic-eucapnic and hyperoxic-hypercapnic steps.

5.2.8   Statistical Analyses

The overnight time series parameters (SaO$_2$, P_{ETCO_2}, and blood measurements) and the sensitivity of the cerebrovascular measurements before and after the nocturnal hypoxic exposures were analyzed using repeated measures analysis of variance (ANOVA). Post hoc tests (Bonferroni) were performed to isolate any significant differences. AMS symptom scores were analyzed by using the non-parametric Freidman test followed by the Dunn's multiple comparison test. Statistical significance was set at $P < 0.05$ for all statistical tests.

5.3   RESULTS

5.3.1   General

All subjects completed the 5 consecutive overnight exposures to hypoxia. The hypoxic environment was well maintained for all subjects throughout the intervention ($F_IO_2 = 13.83\% \pm 0.06$; $F_ICO_2 = 0.0053\% \pm 0.0038$). The majority of subjects reported mild to moderate discomfort during the first hypoxic exposure (mild headache and difficulty sleeping), however these symptoms were ameliorated over the subsequent 4 nights of hypoxia. One subject developed a common cold, which prevented the completion of the acute isocapnic hypoxic protocol immediately following the overnight hypoxic exposures, and was withdrawn from the study; therefore, data from this subject was removed from the final analysis (nocturnal hypoxic intervention, $n = 12$; acute hypoxia and hypercapnia measurements, $n = 11$).

5.3.2   Physiological Responses to the Nocturnal Hypoxic Intervention

Mean SaO_2 values for all subjects during all 5 hypoxic exposures were significantly lower ($P < 0.001$) than SaO_2 measurements recorded during the control sleep (top panel, Figure 1). Mean SaO_2 on the 5th hypoxic exposure was significantly higher when compared to the 1st hypoxic night ($P < 0.001$) and 2nd and 3rd hypoxic exposures ($P < 0.05$).

Figure 5.1

Changes in arterial oxygen saturation (SaO_2) and end-tidal PCO_2 (PET_{CO_2}) throughout the nocturnal hypoxia intervention. Values represent overnight means ± SD. Symbol denotes significantly different than control (CS), or significantly different than exposure 5 (E5) (*$P < 0.05$; *** $P < 0.001$).

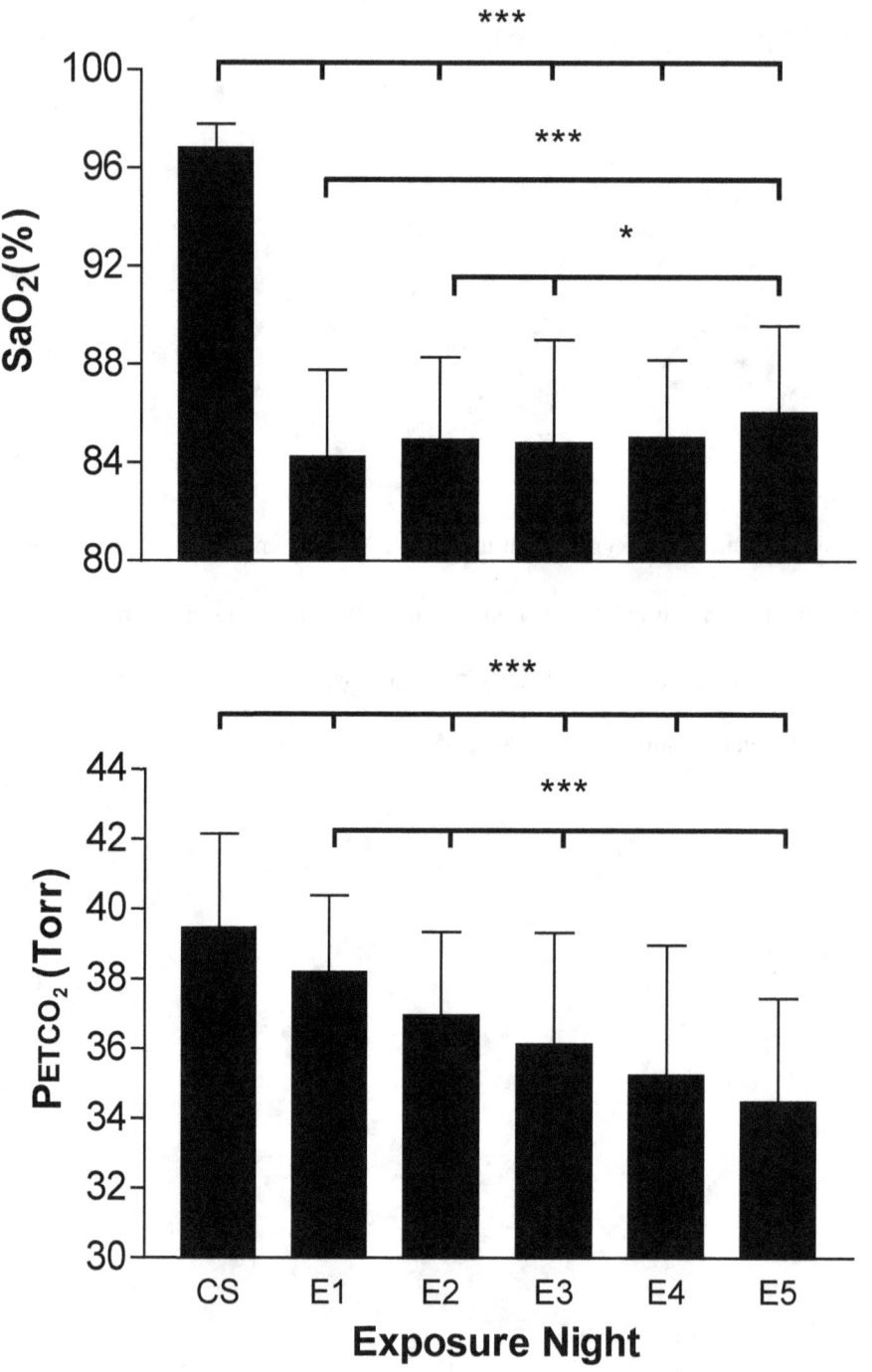

The mean PET_{CO_2} values for all subjects (bottom panel, Figure 1) during each of the overnight hypoxic exposures were significantly lower than control sleep values ($P < 0.001$). Furthermore, the overnight PET_{CO_2} group mean from the 5th hypoxic night was significantly lower than hypoxic nights 1, 2, and 3 ($P < 0.001$).

Mean values for the selected capillary blood samples, which were analyzed immediately before (evening) and at the conclusion (morning) of both the control sleep and all overnight hypoxic exposures, are presented in Figure 2. At the conclusion of eight hours of overnight hypoxia (morning measurements), the capillary partial pressure of O_2 (P_cO_2) values for exposures 1 to 5 were significantly lower than morning P_cO_2 following the control sleep ($P < 0.001$). Similarly, morning capillary partial pressure of CO_2 (P_cCO_2) measurements at the conclusion of exposures 1-5 were significantly lower than the morning after the control sleep P_cCO_2 ($P < 0.001$). Figure 2 illustrates a decline in P_cCO_2 values which persisted between the intermittent hypoxic exposures, with a significant difference observed between evening values (normoxia) at the commencement of the control sleep and prior to exposure 4 ($P < 0.01$). Following 5 days of recovery, P_cCO_2 blood gas measurements had returned to near control values. The hypoxic intervention elicited responses for hemoglobin and hematocrit, illustrated by increasing trends for both evening and morning values (Figure 2). Significant differences were revealed for morning hemoglobin and hematocrit on exposures 3

Figure 5.2

Hematological variability during each of the overnight sessions. CS, control sleep (F_1O_2 = 20.9%), E1-E5, hypoxic exposures (F_1O_2= 13.8%). R5, recovery after five days post intervention. P_cO_2, capillary partial pressure of O_2; P_cCO_2, capillary partial pressure of CO_2. Closed symbols, evening measurements prior to entering chamber; open symbols, morning measurements prior to exiting chamber. Symbol denotes significant difference between evening values against evening control sleep, or significant difference between morning values against morning control sleep. (* $P < 0.05$; ** $P < 0.01$; *** $P < 0.001$).

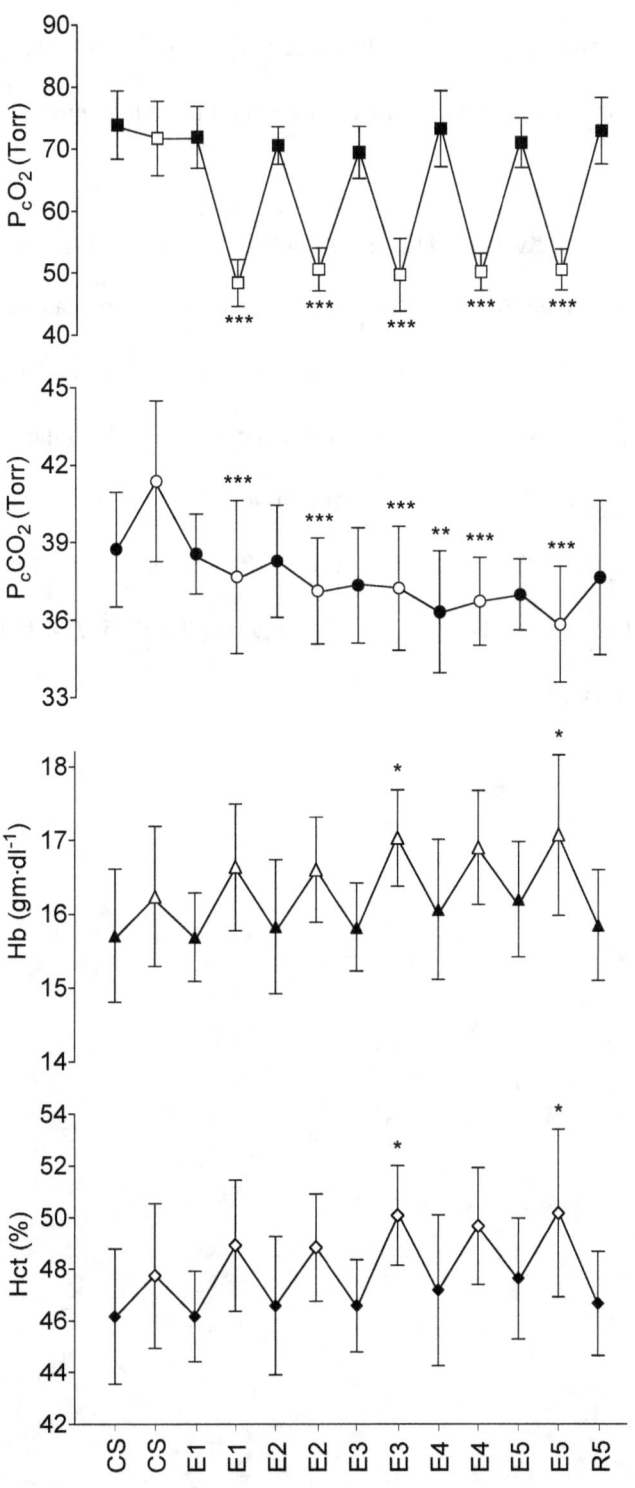

and 5 when compared with the control sleep ($P < 0.05$). Following 5 days of recovery, hemoglobin and hematocrit values had returned to control values.

5.3.3 Symptomatic Responses to the Nocturnal Hypoxic Intervention

The Lake Louise Acute Mountain Sickness Scoring System revealed a significant increase in symptomatology during the 1st and 2nd nights of hypoxic exposure ($P < 0.001$ and $P < 0.01$ respectively) when compared to results from the control sleep (Figure 3). A trend of decreasing symptom severity was observed over the 5 consecutive nights of hypoxia, and the AMS scores on the 1st night were significantly higher than the 3rd, 4th, and 5th nights ($P < 0.05$, $P < 0.01$, and $P < 0.001$ respectively).

Figure 5.3

Changes in acute mountain sickness (AMS) scores throughout the nocturnal hypoxia intervention. AMS scores were assessed as per the consensus on The Lake Louise Acute Mountain Sickness Scoring System (see text for details). CS, control sleep (normoxia); E1-E5, hypoxic exposures (F_IO_2 = 13.8%). Values are means ± SD. Symbol denotes significantly different than control sleep, or significantly different from exposure 1 (E1) (** P < 0.01; *** P < 0.001).

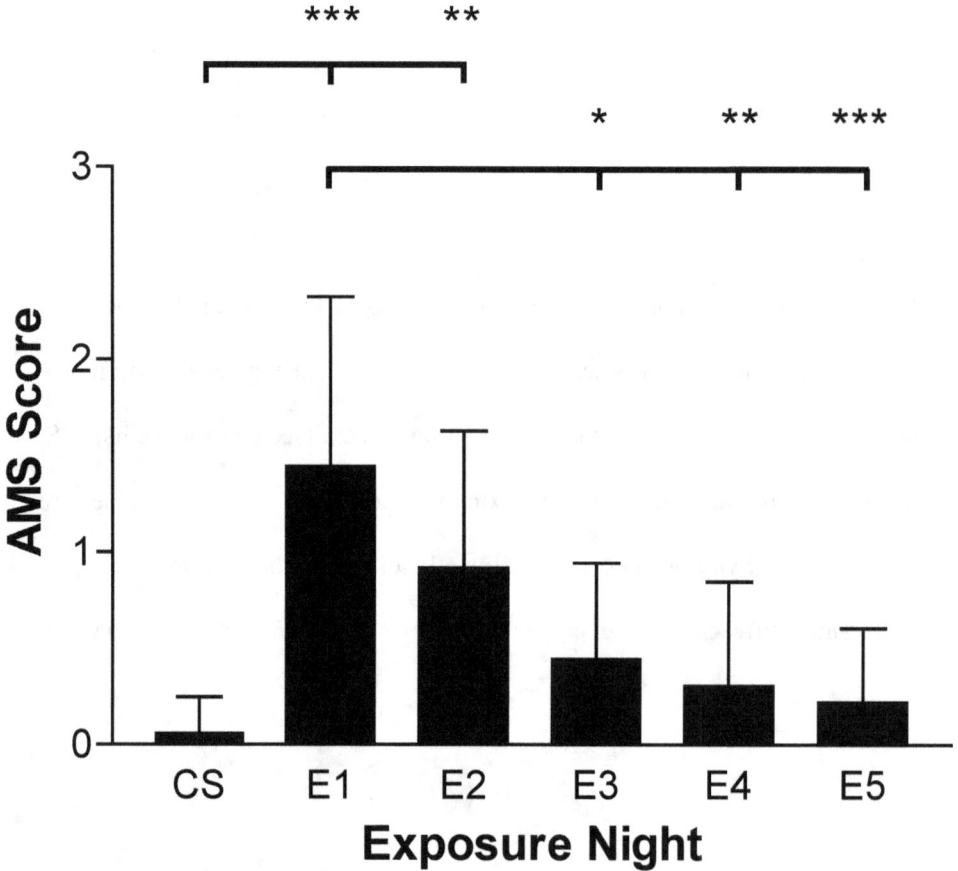

5.3.4   Sensitivity of CBF to Acute Variations in Hypoxia

An example of averaged data for $P_{ET_{O_2}}$ and $P_{ET_{CO_2}}$, measured breath-by-breath,

and $\overline{V_P}$, measured beat-by-beat, during the determination of the CBF response to

acute incremental steps of isocapnic hypoxia is presented in Figure 4. This figure

illustrates that the timing and variation of $P_{ET_{O_2}}$ were well maintained, and that

the levels of $P_{ET_{CO_2}}$ were well controlled at the pre-determined levels. The

degree of the CBF response to the incremental steps of isocapnic hypoxia was

determined by the linear regression between mean values of $\overline{V_P}$ and $100\text{-}SaO_2$.

Figure 5 (top panel) illustrates that the CBF sensitivity to acute variations of

hypoxia significantly increased ($P < 0.01$) from the mean control value (0.35 $\pm$

0.16 cm·s^{-1}·%$^{-1}$) to 0.77 $\pm$ 0.51 cm·s^{-1}·%$^{-1}$ immediately following 5 consecutive

nocturnal hypoxic exposures. Following 5 days of recovery, the sensitivity of

CBF to acute variations in hypoxia returned to near control values.

Figure 5.4

End-tidal PO_2 ($P_{ET_{O_2}}$) and end-tidal PCO_2 ($P_{ET_{CO_2}}$) measured breath-by-breath, regional cerebral oxygen saturation (S_rO_2) measured every 2 s, and mean peak blood velocity ($\overline{V_P}$) measured beat-by-beat during an experimental determination of the cerebrovascular sensitivities to acute variations in hypoxia and CO_2 in one subject (subject ID 0053).   Each symbol represents a 20 s average.

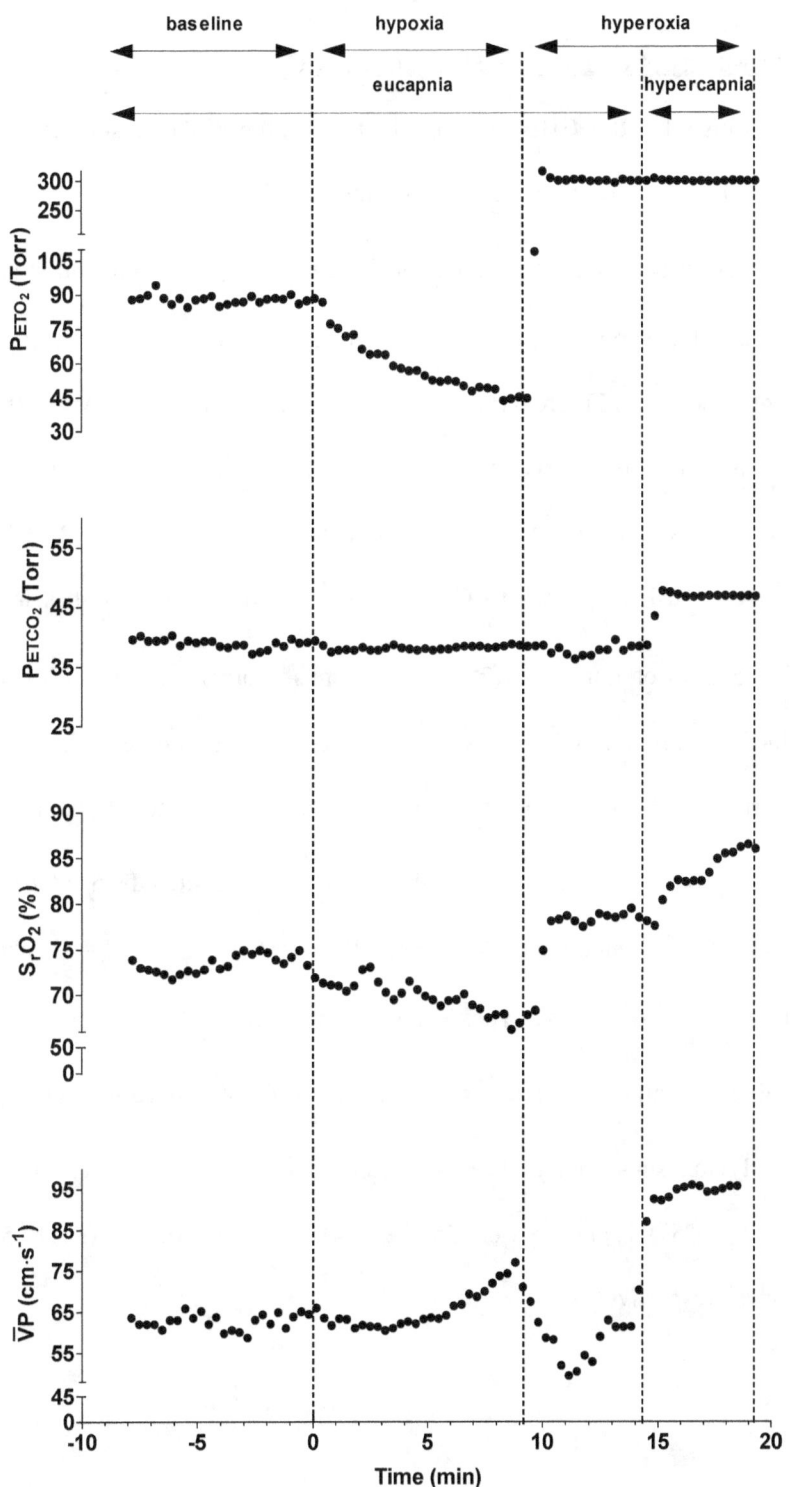

5.3.5   Sensitivity of CBF to Acute Variations in CO_2

Figure 4 illustrates the CBF response to hypercapnia in one subject. The magnitude of the sensitivity of CBF to an acute variation in CO_2 was assessed by linear regression between mean values of $\overline{V}_P$ and P_{ETCO_2} measured during the final minute of eucapnic hyperoxia and hyperoxic hypercapnia. The overall results are presented in Figure 5 (bottom panel). A significant increase ($P < 0.05$) in CBF sensitivity was observed immediately following the hypoxic intervention (3.04 ± 0.74 cm·s^{-1}·Torr^{-1}) compared to mean control measurements (2.23 ± 0.64 cm·s^{-1}·Torr^{-1}). CBF responses to CO_2 subsequently returned to control levels following 5 days of normoxia (2.40 ± 0.81 cm·s^{-1}·Torr^{-1}). Baseline $\overline{V}_P$ was determined by averaging CBF measurements over the final minute of the lead-in period prior to the commencement of the incremental step hypoxic and hypercapnic protocol in order to establish whether $\overline{V}_P$ was altered when the end-tidal gases were regulated at constant levels (P_{ETO_2}=88 Torr; P_{ETCO_2}= 1.5 above the resting values prior to the hypoxic exposures). Immediately following the 5 consecutive overnight hypoxic exposures, baseline $\overline{V}_P$ increased (but not significantly) and subsequently decreased after 5 days of recovery. (Baseline $\overline{V}_P$ (±SD) for C1, C5, R1, and R5 were 55.4 (±10.4), 56.0 (±10.6), 59.6 (±7.9), 53.9 (±8.7) cm·s^{-1}, respectively).

5.3.6   <u>Sensitivity of S_rO_2 to Acute Variations in Hypoxia and CO_2</u>

The S_rO_2 responses to acute variations in hypoxia and CO_2 are illustrated in Figure 4. The determination of S_rO_2 sensitivity to incremental steps of isocapnic hypoxia and hypercapnia were obtained using similar linear regression comparisons that were employed for obtaining CBF sensitivities. While a small increase in the sensitivity of S_rO_2 to the isocapnic hypoxic protocol was observed, no significant differences were revealed between the averaged control measurements, immediately following the hypoxic intervention, and after 5 days of recovery (0.89 ± 0.24 %·%$^{-1}$, 0.93 ± 0.28 %·%$^{-1}$, and 0.88 ± 0.27 %·%$^{-1}$, respectively).   Similarly, no significant differences in S_rO_2 sensitivity to hypercapnia were observed between control days, post hypoxic intervention, and following 5 days of recovery (1.07 ± 0.28 %·Torr^{-1}, 0.94 ± 0.39 %·Torr^{-1}, and 1.21 ± 1.01 %·Torr^{-1} respectively).

Figure 5.5

Top panel: AHR$_{CBF}$, acute cerebral blood flow sensitivity to hypoxia (slope) on control days (C1 and C5), immediately following 5 consecutive overnight exposures of hypoxia (R1), and subsequent recovery (euoxia) five days post intervention (R5). Symbol denotes significantly different from the mean of C1 and C2 (** $P < 0.01$). Bottom panel: AHCR$_{CBF}$, acute cerebral blood flow sensitivity to CO_2. Symbol denotes significantly different from the mean of C1 and C2 (* $P < 0.05$).

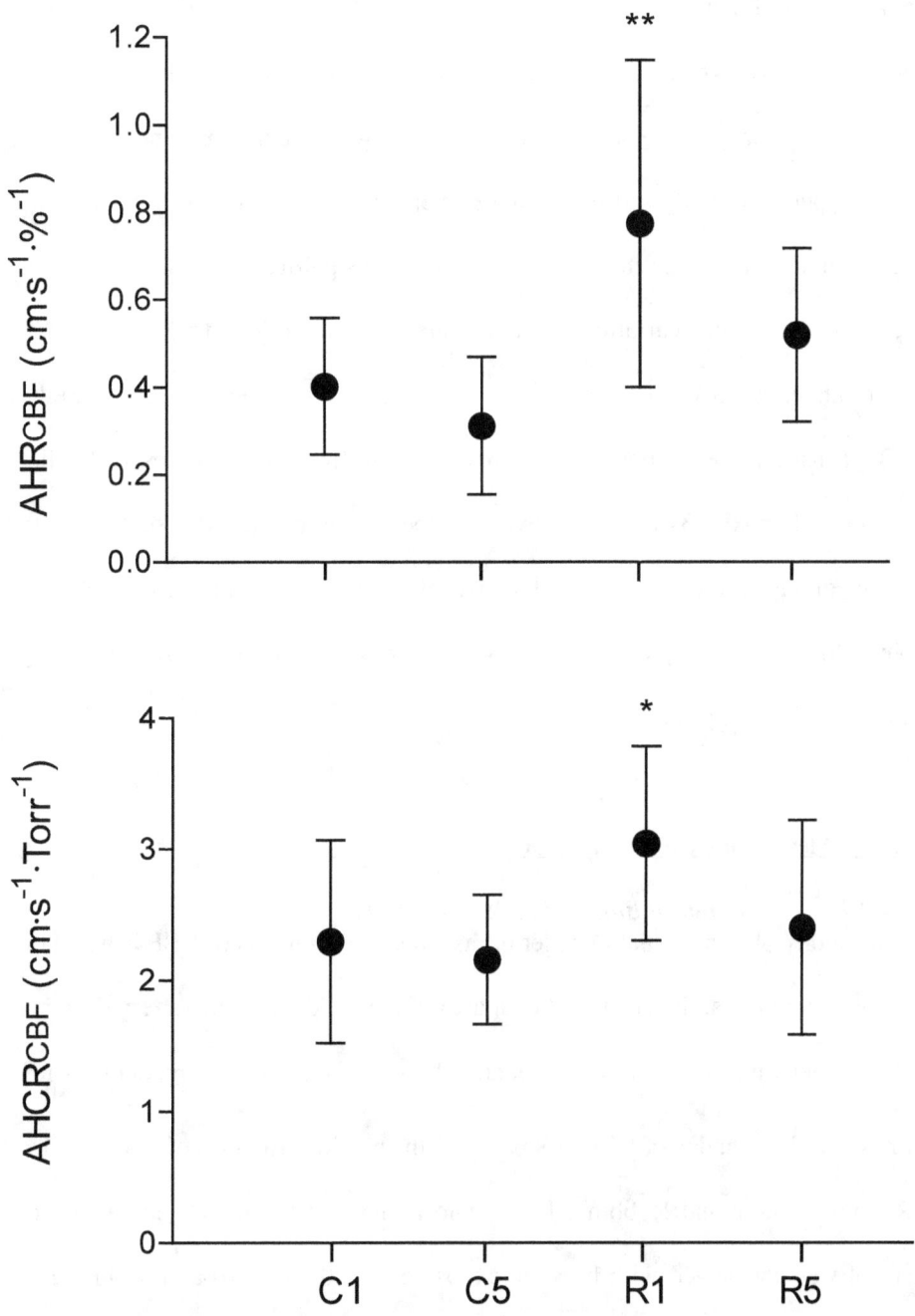

5.4   DISCUSSION

5.4.1   Major Findings

To our knowledge, this study is the first to report on the changes in the cerebrovascular responses to acute exposures of isocapnic hypoxia and hyperoxic hypercapnia following a discontinuous intervention of nocturnal hypoxia. The major findings from this study are that 1) there is a significant increase in the CBF sensitivity to acute variations in isocapnic hypoxia following 5 consecutive overnight exposures of normobaric hypoxia (simulated altitude ~ 4300m); 2) the CBF sensitivity to hyperoxic hypercapnia significantly increases following nocturnal hypoxia; 3) nocturnal hypoxia does not alter the SrO_2 sensitivity to acute variations in O_2 or CO_2; 4) the discontinuous hypoxic intervention elicited physiological and symptomatic responses that are similar to those observed during chronic altitude exposure.

5.4.2   Methodological Considerations

5.4.2.1   Cerebral Blood Flow Measurements
The validity of transcranial Doppler ultrasound measurements of CBF is based on the assumption that the cross sectional area of the middle cerebral artery does not change (Jensen et al., 1996; Poulin et al., 2002). In the present study, our decision to use $\overline{V}_P$ as an index of CBF was based on the previous findings of Poulin and Robbins (Poulin and Robbins, 1996) who found that the total Doppler power signal was unchanged with hypoxic exposures of 20 min (26) and 48 hrs (25).

Furthermore, great care was taken during each measurement to replicate the depth, angle, and position of the insonation pathway as previously reported (Poulin et al., 2002).

5.4.2.2 S_rO_2 *Measurements*

The potential of non-invasive assessments of cerebral oxygenation using near infrared spectroscopy was first described in 1991 as a new monitoring index of oxygen content in the brain (McCormick et al., 1991).   More recently, methodological and comparative studies have validated the accuracy of cerebral oximetry (Kim et al., 2000; Shah et al., 2000).   A stepwise hypoxic protocol, similar to the one used in the present investigation, was implemented by Shah and colleagues (Shah et al., 2000) who compared the performance of the INVOS 4100 cerebral oximeter against direct jugular vein blood gas measurements in humans. Using hypoxic steps of SaO_2 at 95%, 90%, 85%, and 75%, Shah et al. (Shah et al., 2000) reported the overall method comparison analysis (Altman and Bland, 1983) to have a bias (mean value between the differences of the two methods) of −3.1% and precision (standard deviation of the differences) of 12.1%, and concluded that S_rO_2 is a reliable indicator of changes in brain oxygenation induced by hypoxemia.

5.4.2.3   Dynamic Cerebrovascular Measurements in Response to Acute Variations in O_2 and CO_2

The determination of a change in the sensitivity (slope) of cerebrovascular responses following discontinuous or chronic hypoxia, requires a protocol which has high reproducibility within control conditions over time.   Previous observations from our laboratory, using the same protocol as in the present investigation, revealed small coefficients of variation between cerebrovascular measurements in response to acute variations in O_2 and CO_2 (10.4% and 2.9% respectively), while no significant differences were observed between control days (18).

5.4.3   Physiological and Symptomatic Responses to the Nocturnal Hypoxic Exposures

In general, the collective physiological and symptomatic responses observed throughout the nocturnal hypoxic exposures are similar to those observed during chronic high altitude exposures (7, 30, 41). Numerous studies have investigated the impact of discontinuous or intermittent hypoxia on both the ventilatory response to acute hypoxia (Katayama et al., 1999; Rodriguez et al., 1999; Garcia et al., 2000) and the effect on athletic performance (Levine and Stray-Gundersen, 1997; Townsend et al., 2002), whereas there are no previous reports describing the cerebrovascular responses following discontinuous or intermittent hypoxia. Comparisons between the studies mentioned above are somewhat complicated due to the variability of the chosen levels of hypoxia and the duration of the intermittent hypoxic exposures. However, one recent hypoxic intervention utilized by an Australian group (Townsend et al., 2002) consisted of 20 consecutive overnight (8-10 h/night) exposures to a simulated altitude of 2,650m and therefore the first 5 days of their intervention are comparable with our nocturnal hypoxic intervention. Townsend and colleagues (Townsend et al., 2002) reported that PET_{CO_2} was significantly lower ($P < 0.05$) from control values throughout the intervention while the sharpest decline in PET_{CO_2} occurred during the first three nights of hypoxic exposure. In this regard our measurements of PET_{CO_2} (bottom panel, Figure 1) following consecutive bouts of nocturnal hypoxia are in good agreement with those reported by Townsend et al (Townsend et al., 2002).

Intermittent exposure to moderate simulated altitude (5,000m) and extreme simulated altitude (>7,000m) elicits an increased SaO_2 both at rest and during exercise (Richalet et al., 1992; Ricart et al., 2000) as the acclimatization process unfolds. The increases in SaO_2 observed in the present investigation (top panel, Figure 1) are in agreement with those reported by Ricart et al. (Ricart et al., 2000) and Richalet et al. (Richalet et al., 1992), and we concur with these investigators that the increases are primarily a result of ventilatory acclimatization to hypoxia based on respiratory experiments associated with the present study (1). Additionally, a left-shift in the oxyhemoglobin dissociation curve owing to hyperventilation and respiratory alkalosis may have contributed to the rise in SaO_2

throughout the nocturnal hypoxic exposures (Samaja et al., 1986). An alternative mechanism for improved arterial oxygen saturation over the course of nocturnal hypoxia may have been due to a reduction in periodic breathing during sleep, which has been observed in humans under the condition of sustained hypobaric hypoxia (Lahiri et al., 1983).

Turning to the hematology measurements of the present investigation, examination of the top panel in Figure 2 clearly demonstrates the discontinuous nature of the nocturnal hypoxic episodes through the fluctuation between evening and morning measurements of capillary partial pressure of oxygen. Also to note in Figure 2 is the reduction of PCO_2 in the capillary blood over the course of the intervention, which mirrors changes in $P_{ET_{CO_2}}$ illustrated in the bottom panel of Figure 1. Increases in Hct and Hb (Figure 2) are likely a result of hemoconcentration due to hypoxia induced diuresis which has been reported to occur during the early stages of acclimatization to altitude (Singh et al., 1990).

That AMS may develop in humans exposed to simulated altitude (Moore et al., 1986; Savourey et al., 1998) in the natural environment when the altitude gained and rate of ascent is rapid (Singh et al., 1969; Hackett and Rennie, 1976; Basnyat et al., 1999) has been well documented. However in most cases, the symptoms of AMS (headache, nausea, fatigue, and dizziness) are generally self-limiting, and are often ameliorated over 1-2 days if the hypoxic stress is not increased (Hackett and Roach, 2001). In the present study, we observed similar time course changes in AMS symptomatology following discontinuous nocturnal hypoxia, as those reported for both simulated altitude (Moore et al., 1986; Savourey et al., 1998) and chronic altitude exposure in the natural setting (Singh et al., 1969; Hackett and Rennie, 1976; Basnyat et al., 1999).

5.4.4   Cerebrovascular Sensitivities to Acute Variations of Hypoxia and CO_2

Oxygen delivery to the brain is dependent on both oxygen content in the cerebral arteries and CBF. In response to hypoxia, the cerebral circulation also depends on the balance between hypoxemia-induced vasodilatation, and hypocapnia-induced vasoconstriction. Thus, the ventilatory response to hypoxia suggests that CBF should increase and subsequently decrease over days or weeks of chronic hypoxia. Severinghaus and colleagues (Severinghaus et al., 1966) reported the first description of the CBF response during acclimatization to the hypoxia of high altitude. Over the time course of 5 days at an altitude of 3,810m, CBF measurements revealed an abrupt increase (24%) during the initial hours of exposure, followed by a gradual decline that remained 13% above sea level control values on the fifth day. The time domain of this biphasic CBF response to chronic hypoxia in the natural altitude setting has been subsequently supported by others (Otis et al., 1989; Baumgartner et al., 1994; Jensen et al., 1996).

The sensitivity of CBF to acute variations in hypoxia and hypercapnia increases following 5 days of continuous residence at an altitude of 3810m (Jensen et al., 1996). Poulin et al. (Poulin et al., 2002) reported similar increases in sensitivities of CBF following 48hr of continuous isocapnic and poikilocapnic hypoxia in a purpose built chamber. The group from Oxford described a rise of 103% in the CBF sensitivity to acute variations in hypoxia and a rise of 19% in the sensitivity of CBF to an acute variation in CO_2 (Poulin et al., 2002). The major new finding from the present investigation is that discontinuous nocturnal hypoxia elicits similar increases in the sensitivities of CBF to acute variations in hypoxia and CO_2 as has been reported in chronic hypoxia studies. Our data support the observations of Jensen et al. (Jensen et al., 1996) and Poulin et al. (Poulin et al., 2002) in that we found an increase of 116% in the sensitivity of CBF to acute variations in hypoxia, while an increase in 33% was observed in the sensitivity of CBF to acute variations in CO_2.

The sensitivity of S_rO_2 to acute variations in hypoxia and CO_2 did not change following our nocturnal hypoxic protocol. However, individual S_rO_2 values during the dynamic measurements (Figure 4) are representative of those reported in clinical settings (Kim et al., 2000) and in the natural altitude setting (Imray et al., 2000) for equivalent levels of $P_{ET}O_2$ and $P_{ET}CO_2$. The observation that there were no changes in the sensitivity of S_rO_2, and recognizing that S_rO_2 follows changes in systemic oxygen saturation (Kim et al., 2000) suggest that the technique of end-tidal forcing employed for our dynamic measurements was well controlled and that the desired levels of $P_{ET_{O_2}}$ and $P_{ET_{CO_2}}$ were replicated over the different experimental sessions.

In summary, cerebrovascular responses to acute hypoxia and hypercapnia have been measured before and after 5 consecutive nocturnal hypoxic exposures. Our results indicate that discontinuous hypoxia elicits increases in CBF sensitivities to O_2 and CO_2 which are similar to those observed during chronic exposures to hypoxia. While the physiological measurements and symptomatic observations we have reported during the nocturnal hypoxic episodes are similar to the level and time course observed during chronic hypoxia, the time domain for which changes in CBF occur following discontinuous hypoxia remains to be investigated.

5.5   REFERENCES

Ainslie, P. N., Kolb, J. C., Ide, K. and Poulin, M. J. (2003). Effects of 5 nights of normobaric hypoxia on the ventilatory responses to acute hypoxia and hypercapnia. Respiration Physiology and Neurobiology 138: 193-204.

Altman, D. G. and Bland, J. M. (1983). The analysis of method comparison studies. The Statistician 32: 307-317.

Basnyat, B., Lemaster, J. and Litch, J. A. (1999). Everest or bust: a cross sectional, epidemiological study of acute mountain sickness at 4243 meters in the Himalayas. Aviation Space and Environmental Medicine 70(9): 867-73.

Baumgartner, R. W., Bartsch, P., Maggiorini, M., Waber, U. and Oelz, O. (1994). Enhanced cerebral blood flow in acute mountain sickness. Aviation Space and Environmental Medicine 65(8): 726-729.

Buck, A., Schirlo, C., Jasinksy, V., Weber, B., Burger, C., von Schulthess, G. K., Koller, E. A. and Pavlicek, V. (1998). Changes of cerebral blood flow during short-term exposure to normobaric hypoxia. Journal of Cerebral Blood Flow and Metabolism 18(8): 906-10.

Garcia, N., Hopkins, S. R. and Powell, F. L. (2000). Effects of intermittent hypoxia on the isocapnic hypoxic ventilatory response and erythropoiesis in humans. Respiration Physiology 123(1-2): 39-49.

Hackett, P. H. and Rennie, D. (1976). The incidence, importance, and prophylaxis of acute mountain sickness. Lancet 2(7996): 1149-55.

Hackett, P. H. and Roach, R. C. (2001). High-altitude illness. New England
Journal of Medicine 345(2): 107-14.

Howson, M. G., Khamnei, S., McIntyre, M. E., O'Connor, D. F. and Robbins, P.
A. (1987). A rapid computer controlled binary gas mixing system for
studies in respiratory control. Journal of Physiology, London 394: 7P.

Huang, S. Y., Moore, L. G., McCullough, R. E., McCullough, R. G., Micco, A. J.,
Fulco, C., Cymerman, A., Manco-Johnson, M., Weil, J. V. and Reeves, J.
T. (1987). Internal carotid and vertebral arterial flow velocity in men at
high altitude. Journal of Applied Physiology 63(1): 395-400.

Imray, C. H. E., Barnett, N. J., Walsh, S., Clarke, T., Morgan, J., Hale, D., Hoar,
H., Mole, D., Chesner, I. and Wright, A. D. (1998). Near-infrared
spectroscopy in the assessment of cerebral oxygenation at high altitude.
Wilderness and Environmental Medicine 9: 198-203.

Imray, C. H. E., Brearey, S., Clarke, T., Hale, D., Morgan, J., Walsh, S. and
Wright, A. D. (2000). Cerebral oxygenation at high altitude and the
response to carbon dioxide, hyperventilation and oxygen. Clinical Science
98: 159-164.

Jansen, G. F., Krins, A. and Basnyat, B. (1999). Cerebral vasomotor reactivity at
high altitude in humans. Journal of Applied Physiology 86(2): 681-6.

Jensen, J. B., Sperling, B., Severinghaus, J. W. and Lassen, N. A. (1996).
Augmented hypoxic cerebral vasodilation in men during 5 days at 3,810 m
altitude. Journal of Applied Physiology 80(4): 1214-8.

Katayama, K., Sato, Y., Morotome, Y., Shima, N., Ishida, K., Mori, S. and Miyamura, M. (1999). Ventilatory chemosensitive adaptations to intermittent hypoxic exposure with endurance training and detraining. Journal of Applied Physiology 86(6): 1805-11.

Kety, S. S. and Schmidt, C. F. (1948). The effects of altered arterial tensions of carbon dioxide and oxygen on cerebral blood flow and cerebral oxygen consumption of normal young men. Journal of Clinical Investigation 27: 484-492.

Kim, M. B., Ward, D. S., Cartwright, C. R., Kolano, J., Chelhowski, S. and Henson, L. C. (2000). Estimation of Jugular Venous O_2 Saqturation from cerebral oximetry or arterial O_2 saturation during isocapnic hypoxia. Journal of Clinical Monitoring 16: 191-199.

Kolb, J. C., Farran, P., Norris, S., Smith, D. and Mester, J. (2004). Validation of pulse oximetry during progressive normobaric hypoxia utilizing a portable chamber. Canadian Journal of Applied Physiology 29: 3-15.

Lahiri, S., Maret, K. and Sherpa, M. G. (1983). Dependence of high altitude sleep apnea on ventilatory sensitivity to hypoxia. Respiration Physiology 52: 281-301.

Levine, B. D. and Stray-Gundersen, J. (1997). "Living high-training low": effect of moderate-altitude acclimatization with low-altitude training on performance. Journal of Applied Physiology 83(1): 102-12.

McCormick, P. W., Stewart, M., Goetting, M. G. and Balakrishnam, G. (1991). Regional cerebrovascular oxygen saturation by optical spectroscopy in humans. Stroke 22: 596-602.

Moore, L. G., Harrison, G. L., McCullough, R. E., McCullough, R. G., Micco, A. J., Tucker, A., Weil, J. V. and Reeves, J. T. (1986). Low acute hypoxic ventilatory response and hypoxic depression in acute altitude sickness. Journal of Applied Physiology 60(4): 1407-12.

Otis, S. M., Rossman, M. E., Schneider, P. A., Rush, M. P. and Ringelstein, E. B. (1989). Relationship of cerebral blood flow regulation to acute mountain sickness. Journal of Ultrasound in Medicine 8(3): 143-8.

Poulin, M. J., Fatemian, M., Tansley, J. G., O'Connor, D. F. and Robbins, P. A. (2002). Changes in cerebral blood flow during and after 48 h of both isocapnic and poikilocapnic hypoxia in humans. Experimental Physiology 87.5: 633-642.

Poulin, M. J. and Robbins, P. A. (1996). Indexes of flow and cross-sectional area of the middle cerebral artery using Doppler ultrasound during hypoxia and hypercapnia in humans. Stroke 27: 2244-2250.

Ricart, A., Casas, H., Casas, M., Pages, T., Palacios, L., Rama, R., Rodriguez, F. A., Viscor, G. and Ventura, J. L. (2000). Acclimatization near home? Early respiratory changes after short-term intermittent exposure to simulated altitude. Wilderness and Environmental Medicine 11(2): 84-8.

Richalet, J. P., Bittel, J., Herry, J. P., Savourey, G., Le Trong, J. L., Auvert, J. F. and Janin, C. (1992). Use of a hypobaric chamber for pre-acclimatization before climbing Mount Everest. International Journal of Sports Medicine 13(Suppl 1): S216-20.

Roach, R. C., Bartsch, P., Hackett, P. H. and Olez, O. (1993). The Lake Louise Acute Mountain Sickness Scoring System. In: *Hypoxia and Mountain Medicine*. J. R. Sutton, C. S. Houston and G. Coates. Burlington, VT, Queen City Press: 272-274.

Roach, R. C. and Hackett, P. H. (2001). Frontiers of hypoxia research: acute mountain sickness. Experimental Biology 204: 3161-3170.

Robbins, P. A., Swanson, G. D. and Howson, M. G. (1982). A prediction correction scheme for forcing alveolar gases along certain time courses. Journal of Applied Physiology 52: 1353-1357.

Rodriguez, F. A., Casas, H., Casas, M., Pages, T., Rama, R., Ricart, A., Ventura, J. L., Ibanez, J. and Viscor, G. (1999). Intermittent hypobaric hypoxia stimulates erythropoiesis and improves aerobic capacity. Medicine and Science in Sports and Exercise 31(2): 264-8.

Saito, S., Nishihara, F., Takazawa, T., Kanai, M., Aso, C., Shiga, T. and Shimada, H. (1999). Exercise-induced cerebral deoxygenation among untrained trekkers at moderate altitudes. Archives of Environmental Health 54(4): 271-277.

Samaja, M., di Prampero, P. E. and Cerretelli, P. (1986). The role of 2.3-DPG in the oxygen transport at altitude. Respiration Physiology 64: 191.

Savourey, G., Caterini, R., Launay, J. C., Guinet, A., Besnard, Y., Hanniquet, A. M. and Bittel, J. (1998). Positive end expiratory pressure as a method for preventing acute mountain sickness. European Journal of Applied Physiology 77(1-2): 32-6.

Schoene, R. B. (1999). The brain at high altitude. Wilderness and Environmental Medicine 10(2): 93-6.

Severinghaus, J. W. (1979). Simple, accurate equations for human blood O2 dissociation computations. Journal of Applied Physiology 46(3): 599-602.

Severinghaus, J. W. (2001). Cerebral circulation at high altitude. *In: High Altitude: An Exploration of Human Adaptation*. T. F. Hornbein, Schoene, R. B. New York, Marcel Dekker, Inc. 161: 343-375.

Severinghaus, J. W., Chiodi, H., Eger, E., Brandstater, B. and Hornbein, T. F. (1966). Cerebral blood flow in man at high altitude. Circulation Research 19: 274-282.

Shah, N., Trivedi, N. K., Clack, S. L., Shah, M., Shah, P. P. and Barker, S. (2000). Impact of hypoxemia on the performance of cerebral oximeter in volunteer subjects. Journal of Neurosurgical Anesthesiology 12(3): 201-209.

Singh, I., Khanna, P. K., Lai, M., Roy, S. B. and Subramanyam, C. S. (1969). Acute mountain sickness. New England Journal of Medicine 280(4): 175-184.

Singh, M. V., Rawal, S. B. and Tyagi, A. K. (1990). Body fluid status on induction, reinduction and prolonged stay at high altitude on human volunteers. International Journal of Biometeorology 34: 93-97.

Townsend, N., Gore, C., Hahn, A., McKenna, M., Aughey, R., Clark, S., Kinsman, T., Hawley, J. and Chow, C. (2002). Living high-training low increases hypoxic ventilatory response of well-trained endurance athletes. Journal of Applied Physiology 93: 149-1505.

CHAPTER 6

GENERAL DISCUSSION

6.0   SYNOPSIS OF FINDINGS

The studies described in the present Thesis were designed to provide an in-depth physiological and symptomatic insight into the effects of intermittent normobaric hypoxia using portable chambers. This Thesis makes a unique contribution in that there have been few systematic investigations that have adumbrated the potential benefits, and or risks, associated with consecutive overnight hypoxic exposures using the commercially available chambers.

In the first results chapter (Chapter 2), a method comparison investigation considered the validity of non-invasive pulse oximetry measurements of oxygen saturation (SpO_2) with direct arterial oxygen saturation (SaO_2) measurements via co-oximetry. Validation of pulse oximetry in commercially available normobaric hypoxic chambers had not been previously reported. Over 2.5 hrs, the inspired fraction of oxygen inside the chamber was progressively reduced from 20.9% to 11.5%. Measurements of SaO_2 throughout the progressive hypoxic exposure were compared with SpO_2 estimates of oxygen saturation using reflectance and transmission pulse oximetry sensors. Regression analysis and methods for assessing agreement between SaO_2 and SpO_2 were similar when all of the data was compared. However, when $SaO_2 < 85\%$, the reflectance sensors exhibited greater validity than the transmission sensors. The major conclusions from this study were firstly that pulse oximeters provide reasonable accuracy for estimating SaO_2 during normobaric hypoxic exposures when the SaO_2 is greater than 85%.

However, the accuracy of the pulse oximetry devices used in this experiment deteriorated at lower levels of hypoxemia. Secondly, the reflectance sensor provided greater validity than the transmission sensor when compared to direct measurements of SaO_2.

In light of these findings, caution should be exercised when monitoring individuals with pulse oximetry during de-saturation episodes below 85%. From a practical perspective, pulse oximetry provides reliable monitoring of hypoxemia at rest when the fraction of inspired oxygen range is between 20.9% and approximately 14%. This practical relevance was important in designing the overnight hypoxic intervention described in Chapters 4 and 5, to ensure the health status of the subjects, and to obtain accurate estimations of systemic oxygenation.

To address changes in respiratory control and alterations in cerebrovascular dynamics that may occur following intermittent normobaric hypoxia, it was essential to first develop a protocol having high reproducibility of measurements during control experiments. To be effective, such a protocol would need to consist of several levels of hypoxia in which the time spent at each level was long enough for both the ventilatory and cerebrovascular responses to unfold, but short enough to prevent the development of hypoxic ventilatory decline (HVD). In previous work, Mou and collegues (1994) reported that a protocol which consisted of 50 s at seven levels of hypoxia resulted in ventilatory responses which did not result in HVD. However, Poulin and Robbins (1996) indicated that 50 s may be too short for the cerebrovascular responses to occur.

Therefore, in Chapter 3 a protocol is described for determining the acute cerebrovascular and ventilatory responses to hypoxia and hypercapnia, which accounted for the time sensitive characteristics of both physiological variables.

The main finding from the study described in Chapter 3 was that by extending the protocol of Mou et al. (1995) from 50 s to 90 s, both cerebrovascular and ventilatory responses to hypoxia and hypercapnia were measured without any indication of HVD. Paired t-tests of the acute measurements revealed no significant differences, thus illustrating that the cerebrovascular and ventilatory sensitivities to hypoxia and hypercapnia were similar on the two separate experimental testing days. Furthermore the low coefficients of variation advocated strong day-to-day reproducibility of the outcome variables in this protocol.

Turning towards practical considerations of the protocol, it is noteworthy that the process of acclimatization to hypoxia is associated with changes in ventilation (Basu et al., 1996; Tansley et al., 1998) and cerebral blood flow (CBF) (Jensen et al., 1996; Poulin et al., 2002). However the potential role that changes in CBF may have on the ventilatory acclimatization to hypoxia, or the etiology of diseases such as acute mountain sickness (AMS) and high altitude cerebral edema remains unclear (Roach and Hackett, 2001). In light of the findings from Chapter 3, which indicated the protocol was well suited to quantify the cerebrovascular and ventilatory responses to acute hypoxia, the protocol may help further elucidate the role of changes in CBF and ventilatory acclimatization to chronic or intermittent hypoxia, and may further provide insight to the pathology of altitude related illnesses.

The next scope of the work described in Chapters 4 and 5 respectively, addresses the issues of alterations in respiratory control and cerebrovascular responses to the acute hypoxic protocol presented in Chapter 3, both before and after an intermittent normobaric hypoxic intervention. Twelve young adults participated in these studies. In brief, the intervention design was as follows: Each subject slept 8 h/day overnight for 5 consecutive days in purpose-designed normobaric hypoxic chambers at a simulated altitude of 4300m. Subjects entered the chambers at approximately 2300 hrs and exited at 0700 hrs the following morning. Between the nocturnal hypoxic exposures, subjects maintained their normal daily activities.

In Chapter 4, the following specific hypothesis was tested: That five consecutive nocturnal hypoxic exposures would elicit similar changes in the acute hypoxic ventilatory response (AHVR) and acute hypercapnic ventilatory response

(AHCVR) as has been reported following chronic hypoxic exposures. The results from Chapter 4 yielded two important and novel findings. Firstly, five overnight episodes of normobaric hypoxia elicited a pronounced increase in AHVR and leftward shift of the AHCVR, together with an increase in the slope of this relationship. Secondly, the significant decrease in $P_{ET_{CO_2}}$ throughout the nocturnal hypoxic intervention correlated both with the leftward shift and increase in the slope of the AHCVR, and has not previously been reported following intermittent hypoxic exposures.

Consistent with the hypothesis presented in Chapter 4, these results indicate that five consecutive nights of normobaric hypoxia elicit similar modifications in respiratory control as those reported in response to chronic hypoxia. The major reason why previous intermittent studies (Katayama et al., 1998) and chamber studies (Howard and Robbins, 1995; Tansely et al., 1998) have not shown changes in the AHCVR are most likely due to the level of hypoxia being too mild and/or the duration of exposure being too short.

The effect of intermittent hypoxia on cerebrovascular regulation in humans has not been previously reported. Alterations in cerebrovascular sensitivities following the overnight hypoxic intervention are presented in Chapter 5. As well, hematological and symptoms associated with AMS were characterized during each of the overnight exposures. The technique of end-tidal forcing (Chapter 3) was used to examine CBF and regional cerebral oxygen saturation (S_rO_2) responses to acute variations in O_2 and CO_2 twice prior to, immediately after, and 5 days following the overnight hypoxic exposures. Transcranial Doppler ultrasound was used to assess CBF, and near infrared spectroscopy was used to assess S_rO_2. Throughout the nocturnal hypoxic exposures, end-tidal PCO_2 decreased ($P < 0.001$) while arterial oxygen saturation increased ($P < 0.001$) compared with overnight normoxic control measurements. Symptoms associated with AMS were significantly greater than control values on the 1st night ($P < 0.001$) and 2nd night ($P < 0.01$) of nocturnal hypoxia. Immediately following the nocturnal hypoxic intervention, the sensitivity of CBF to acute variations in O_2 and CO_2 increased 116% ($P < 0.01$) and 33% ($P < 0.05$), respectively, when compared with control values; no changes in the sensitivity of S_rO_2 were observed.

The results presented in Chapter 5 are novel and important in that they represent the first measurements of cerebrovascular responses to intermittent hypoxia. The major finding from this study is that five consecutive overnight exposures of normobaric hypoxia elicits a significant increase in CBF sensitivity to acute alterations of O_2 and CO_2. Interestingly the changes in CBF sensitivities reported in Chapter 5 are consistent with those reported for chronic exposures to hypoxia during sojourns to altitude (Severinghaus et al., 1966; Otis et al., 1989; Jensen et al., 1996). One possible explanation for the similar CBF changes following intermittent and chronic hypoxia supports the postulate of Neubauer (2001) that the consecutive intermittent hypoxic exposures engendered a cumulative effect over time.

Acclimatization to hypoxia, which generally occurs over days to weeks, develops through multiple responses by different systems of the body, which mitigate the reduction of oxygen at the tissue level. The most important responses include; 1) increased ventilation stimulated by both peripheral and central chemoreceptors, and 2) improvement in blood oxygen content via hematogenesis. As observed in Chapter 5, the process of acclimatization was progressing in sequential steps following each hypoxic exposure. Successive increases in SaO_2, reductions in $P_{ET}CO_2$ which occurred secondary to hyperventilation, and elevated hematocrit and hemoglobin concentrations, collectively provide evidence that the process of acclimatization to intermittent hypoxia was unfolding. These physiological perturbations are in concert with the alterations in respiratory control detailed in Chapter 4.

An additional important finding from Chapter 5 indicates that the symptoms of AMS (headache, nausea, malaise, dizziness, and difficulty sleeping) peaked during the initial hypoxic episode and were subsequently ameliorated over the course of the intermittent hypoxic intervention. These changes in AMS symptomatology occurred in a similar time frame as the systemic oxygenation improved and SaO_2 increased. The reduction in AMS support the hypothesis that the optimal dose of hypoxia required to stimulate beneficial physiologic and symptomatic changes requires adequate recovery (Levine and Stray-Gunderson, 1997). Alternatively, the mechanism for improved oxygen content over the course of the intermittent hypoxic exposures may have been due to a reduction in periodic breathing during sleep, which has been observed during residence at altitude (Lahiri et al., 1983).

It is concluded from the completion of the studies in Chapters 2, 3, 4, and 5 that the objectives of this thesis have been realized. A critical comparison between the non-invasive measurements of oxygen saturation with direct blood measurements revealed that pulse oximetry is a reliable method to monitor levels of hypoxemia during mild to moderate exposures of normobaric hypoxia. Subsequently, in order to establish a method for the quantification of cerebrovascular and ventilatory responses to acute variations in O_2 and CO_2 a sophisticated protocol was designed utilizing the technique of end-tidal forcing. This protocol was successful in replicating measurements in control subjects overtime, and therefore was deemed capable of quantifying alterations in cerebrovascular and ventilatory sensitivities arising from chronic or intermittent hypoxic exposures. An intervention consisting of five consecutive overnight normobaric hypoxic exposures was then implemented, and the protocol was used to determine the extent and time frame for the development and reversibility of physiological and symptomatic modifications.

6.2   CONCLUSIONS

From the studies described above, the main conclusions are that an intermittent normobaric hypoxic intervention, consisting of five consecutive overnight exposures to a simulated altitude of 4300m, elicits perturbations in the acute cerebrovascular and ventilatory responses to both hypoxia and hypercapnia, which are similar to changes following chronic altitude exposure.   Individual variability to intermittent hypoxia may have an impact on the rate at which the process of acclimatization proceeds.   The extent of physiological and symptomatic responses to intermittent hypoxia are likely to be associated with the severity of hypoxia as well as the length and number of recurrent episodes of hypoxia.

6.3   RECOMMENDATIONS FOR FUTURE WORK

From conducting the investigations in the present thesis and from reviewing the literature, the following directions for future work are proposed in the area of intermittent hypoxia.

First, it would seem important to investigate further the time domain during which alterations in cerebrovascular and ventilatory manifestations unfold following recurrent episodes of hypoxia. While much is known regarding the time course of ventilatory acclimatization hypoxia, there is little information concerning the rate of change in cerebrovascular responses following intermittent hypoxia. Characterizing theses serial time changes may be beneficial to better understand the risks associated with the pathophysiology of altitude-related illnesses. In this regard, studies are warranted which quantify the progression of responses following each overnight hypoxic episode, during an extended (~2 weeks) intermittent hypoxic intervention. Furthermore, the reversibility of these changes should be assessed during a similar time course of recovery. Alternatively, interventions consisting of shorter intermittent hypoxic exposures (2-3 h·day^{-1}) have the potential to assist in determining how the 'dose' of repeated hypoxic exposures influences the threshold for change.

Interest in the affects of chronic intermittent hypoxia of short duration (60 – 90 s) is clinically relevant in discerning the pathophysiology of sleep-related breathing disorders. Interpretation of the cerebrovascular and ventilatory responses to acute variations in hypoxia and hypercapnia, in individuals exhibiting recurrent episodes of hypoxia during sleep, may therefore be important in understanding the association between obstructive sleep apnea and stroke.

The vast majority of protocols employed to address ventilatory and cerebrovascular sensitivities to acute hypoxia, incorporate methods which control the level of PE_{TCO_2} to reflect the subjects resting values (i.e. isocapnia). However, as the ventilatory acclimatization to hypoxia proceeds, PE_{TCO_2} levels fall resulting in respiratory alkalosis. Therefore, acute responses to hypoxia following chronic or intermittent hypoxic exposures may require the development of a poikilocapnic protocol, which allows alterations of PE_{TCO_2} to fall naturally throughout the experiment while pulmonary ventilation increases. The discernment between poikilocapnic and isocapnic tests of hypoxic ventilatory responses following acclimatization to hypoxia have not been previously investigated.

Finally, limited data exist concerning the direct comparison between the effects of chronic hypoxia vs. intermittent hypoxia. Instituting a repeated measures design, where each subject partakes in both chronic and intermittent hypoxic interventions, may help determine the extent to which the treatments are similar or whether they result in different levels of acclimatization.

It is envisaged that conducting further research in the areas outlined above will lead to a greater understanding of the physiological and symptomatic responses associated with intermittent hypoxia. Furthermore, these studies should contribute to the body of knowledge exploring the complex inter-relationship of variables which govern the process of acclimatization to hypoxia.

REFERENCES

Basu, C. K., Selvamurthy, W., Bhaumick, G., Gautam, R. K. and Sawhney, R. C. (1996). Respiratory changes during initial days of acclimatization to increasing altitudes. Aviation Space and Environmental Medicine 67: 40-5.

Howard, L.S.G.E. and Robbins, P.A., 1995. Alterations in respiratory control during eight hours of isocapnic and poikilocapnic hypoxia in humans. Journal of Applied Physiology 78, 1098-1107.

Jensen, J. B., Sperling, B., Severinghaus, J. W. and Lassen, N. A. (1996). Augmented hypoxic cerebral vasodilation in men during 5 days at 3,810 m altitude. Journal of Applied Physiology 80: 1214-8.

Katayama, K., Sato, Y., Morotome, Y., Shima, N., Ishida, K., Mori, S. and Miyamura, M. (1999). Ventilatory chemosensitive adaptations to intermittent hypoxic exposure with endurance training and detraining. Journal of Applied Physiology 86: 1805-11.

Lahiri, S., Maret, S. and Sherpa, M.G. (1983). Dependence of high altitude sleep apnea on ventilatory sensitivity to hypoxia. Respiration Physiology 52: 281-301.

Levine, B. D. and Stray-Gunderson, J. (1997). High altitude training and competition. In: The Team Physician's Handbook. Mellion, M. B., Walsh, M. W. and Shelton, L. G. St. Louis, Hanley and Belfus, Inc. 186-193.

Mou, X. B., Howard, L. S. and Robbins, P. A. (1995). A protocol for determining the shape of the ventilatory response to hypoxia in humans. Respiration Physiology 101: 139-43.

Neubauer, J. (2001). Physiological and pathophysiological responses to intermittent hypoxia. Journal of Applied Physiology 90: 1593-1599.

Otis, S. M., Rossman, M. E., Schneider, P. A., Rush, M. P. and Ringelstein, E. B. (1989). Relationship of cerebral blood flow regulation to acute mountain sickness. Journal of Ultrasound in Medicine 8: 143-8.

Poulin, M. J. and Robbins, P. A. (1996). Indexes of flow and cross-sectional area of the middle cerebral artery using Doppler ultrasound during hypoxia and hypercapnia in humans. Stroke 27: 2244-2250.

Poulin, M. J., Fatemian, M., Tansley, J. G., O'Connor, D. F. and Robbins, P. A. (2002). Changes in cerebral blood flow during and after 48 h of both isocapnic and poikilocapnic hypoxia in humans. Experimental Physiology 87.5: 633-642.

Roach, R. and Hackett, P. H. (2001). Frontiers of hypoxia research: acute mountain sickness. The Journal of Experimental Biology 204: 3161-3170.

Severinghaus, J. W., Chiodi, H., Eger, E., Brandstater, B. and Hornbein, T. F. (1966). Cerebral blood flow in man at high altitude. Circulation Research 19: 274-282.

Tansley, J. G., Fatemian, M., Howard, L. S., Poulin, M. J. and Robbins, P. A. (1998). Changes in respiratory control during and after 48 h of isocapnic and poikilocapnic hypoxia in humans. Journal of Applied Physiology 85(6): 2125-34.

PUBLICATIONS ASSOCIATED WITH THIS THESIS

Kolb, J. C., Farran P., Norris, S. R., Smith, D. and Mester, J. (2004). Validation of pulse oximetry during progressive normobaric hypoxia utilizing a portable chamber. Canadian Journal of Applied Physiology 29(1): 3-15.

Ainslie, P. N.[1], Kolb, J. C. [1], Ide, K. and Poulin, M. J. (2003). Effects of 5 nights of normobaric hypoxia on the ventilatory responses to acute hypoxia and hypercapnia. Respiration Physiology and Neurobiology 138: 193-204.

Kolb, J. C., Ainslie, P. N., Ide, K. and Poulin, M. J. (2004). Protocol for determining the acute cerebrovascular and ventilatory responses to incremental step changes of isocapnic hypoxia in humans. Respiration Physiology and Neurobiology 141: 191-199.

Kolb, J. C., Ainslie, P. N., Ide, K. and Poulin, M. J. (2004). Effects of 5 consecutive nocturnal hypoxic exposures on the cerebrovascular responses to acute hypoxia and hypercapnia in humans. Journal of Applied Physiology 96: 1745-1754.

---

[1] Both authors made an equal contribution to this paper.

Kolb, J. C., Ainslie, P. N., Ide, K. and Poulin, M. J. Effects of 5 consecutive nocturnal hypoxic exposures on respiratory control and hematogenesis in humans. *In: Post-Genomic Perspectives in Modeling and Control of Breathing*. Advances in Experimental Medicine and Biology. (In Press)

PUBLISHED ABSTRACTS

Kolb, J. C. (1997). Hyperbaric prophylaxis of acute mountain sickness. In: Hypoxia: Women at Altitude; Proceedings of the Tenth International Hypoxia Symposium at Lake Louise, Canada, edited by C. S. Houston and G. Coates. P. 316.

Kolb, J. C., Norris, S. R., Smith, D., Henderson, J. and Hillis, F. (2001). Intermittent normobaric hypoxia enhances acclimation. High Alt. Med. Biol. 2:105.

Kolb, J. C., Norris, S. R., Neil, R., Hillis, F. and Smith, D. (2001). Acclimation to intermittent normobaric hypoxia ameliorates acute mountain sickness. *In: Perspectives and Profiles; Book of Abstracts, 6th Annual Congress of the European College of Sport Science*. Cologne, Germany, edited by J. Mester, G. King, H. Strüder. p. 1084.

Kolb, J. C., Ainslie, P. N., Ide, K. and Poulin, M. J. (2002). A protocol for determining the cerebrovascular and ventilatory responses to incremental step changes of isocapnic hypoxia. High Alt. Med. Biol. 3:441.

Kolb, J.C., P. Farran, S. Norris, and D. Smith (2002). Validation of pulse oximetry during progressive normobaric hypoxia utilizing a portable chamber. High Alt. Med. Biol. 3:453.

COMMUNICATIONS TO SCHOLARLY MEETINGS

Kolb, J. C. Intermittent normobaric hypoxia enhances acclimation.
12ʰ International Hypoxia Symposium, Jasper, Alberta, Canada, March 10-14, 2001.